Institute
©1970

Wine Institute, 717 Market

July 22, 1970

C O N T E N T S

S.P. LUCIA

Wine
and the
Digestive
System

Dedicated to all those
past and present who have contributed to
the knowledge of the essential and marvelous
ingredients of wine—which from the beginning
of history has been man's adequate
companion to bread.

Wine
and the
Digestive
System

*The Effects of Wine and its
Constituents on the Organs and
Functions of the Gastrointestinal Tract*

A Selected Annotated Bibliography by
Salvatore Pablo Lucia, M.D.

Fortune House
San Francisco

Wine and the Digestive System

Table of Contents

Introduction

The present monograph is part of a major bibliographic effort dealing with an assembly of references relative to the effect of wine and its constituents on the major organ systems of the human body. Originally, the bibliography was gathered in an attempt to trace the history of wine as part of the history of medicine. As this project grew in scope and size, it became clear that wine has a cultural lineage parallel with that of recorded history since it has been used as a food, as a medicine and as a menstruum for other therapeutic agents, as well as an important element in religious and social life. The literature on wine, waxing and waning through diverse cultural epochs, forms a continuous thread until the fateful era of American Prohibition early in the twentieth century when, at least in the United States, prejudiced silence imposed its reign for a generation.

During Prohibition, the use of alcoholic beverages was seriously hampered and research on beverage alcohol was temporarily suppressed. As a consequence, the medical lore of wine and the scientific documentation of its varied physiological effects became buried in serious bias. A generation grew up which learned to know wine only as a pleasant and economical drink containing alcohol—hardly realizing that it is a biologic fluid of unusual complexity as well as one of the oldest known medicinal and dietary beverages.

Wine is the naturally fermented juice of the grape containing all of its virtues and essences. Always subject to continuous and infinite biologic change, wine enjoys a temporal life span, during which it is drinkable, followed by a natural decline. This unusual aspect is most significant, saporifically and functionally, at the height of its maturity.

Not only the grapes, their stems, pips and skins, but also the soil in which the vines are grown share in proportion the aroma, bouquet, and chemical composition of the finished product.

The must, containing the substance of the grape, its vine and the derivatives of the soil, undergoes chemical changes during fermentation which result in a wide range of biologically active constituents—alcohols, acids, aldehydes, ethereal substances, esters, polyhydroxyphenols, anthocyanins, nitrogenous compounds, enzymes, vitamins, and traces of carbohydrates. In addition, one finds inorganic constituents—minerals, acids, and salts.

The aroma and bouquet of wine, important to all who enjoy it, are the result of the aromatic ensemble created by the aldehydes, esters, volatile and fixed acids, and other substances yet to be defined, which are released during fermentation and remain viable for the life of the wine. The ultimate characteristic of a wine is that of the grape of its origin (e.g., Pinot Noir, Cabernet Sauvignon, etc.).

One of the earliest uses of wine was as a nutrient—it supplies calories, vitamins and minerals. In medicine, wine has been used both as menstruum and healing agent. The medicinal use of wine remained purely empirical until chemical analysis and laboratory studies divulged its physiologic effects. Pharmacodynamically, the most important constituents of wine are: ethyl alcohol, many aldehydes, organic acids, carbohydrates, and anthocyanins. It should be stated here that although the pharmacodynamic action of some of the single constituents of wine is known, the total effect of wine transcends the effect of its single components.

An important use of wine concerns its sedative propensity—a quality abundantly endorsed in medical writings, ancient and modern. The sedative effect is apparently due to the interaction between aldehydes in balance with alcohol and other ethereal substances. The coloring matters derived from the skin of the grape, the anthocyanins, are responsible for some of the antibiotic effect of wine—a property known to ancient cultures and still exploited by the peoples of the Mediterranean who mix wine with water in order to render the latter more potable.

Wine is of value in certain metabolic diseases such as diabetes, where it exerts a stabilizing effect on the level of blood sugar concentration. The mechanism of this action is not clear, but it has been suggested that the sugar (d-fructose) of wine is more rapidly absorbed than glucose, thus neutralizing significant elevations of the latter sugar in the blood.

Observations of the beneficial effects of wine have provided the necessary impetus to collect data for this annotated genealogy of wine. Eventually, the author hopes to present a series of monographs describing the effects of wine on all organ systems of the human body. The digestive system has taken precedence over other equally important systems because of its obvious primary exposure to wine as an aliment. But more than that, the digestive system shares importance with the reproductive system in the quest for survival. The role of wine as an element of survival becomes apparent when it is realized that man knew wine as a food before he used it as a medicine and as an element in his spiritual practices.

Beyond a bibliographer's love for the recondite and a scientist's love for laboratory techniques, what is the purpose of this monograph on wine? Notably, to acquaint the physician with the literature on a socio-cultural substance in continuous use since the earliest recorded history; to guide the interested reader through an important facet of medical lore as well as to illustrate that the medicinal use of wine preceded by millenia the scientific proof of its value; to permit an objective evaluation of the role of wine as nutrient and medicine; and finally, to supply the scientific evidence essential to move those whose bias rules their thinking. With these objectives in mind, the references have been arranged chronologically, so that an historical perspective could be achieved which would indicate the transition from the empirical and conjectural to the precise and scientific. In addition, this arrangement illustrates the sapience and continuity of perceptive clinical thinking. The author also must admit to making particular use of this publication as an opportunity to acquaint the reader with some of the therapeutic uses of wine, within the scope of this monograph, with the hope that some further thought and action might be stimulated in this very important area.

In keeping with standards set by anatomical texts, this presentation is divided into seven sections, each one dealing with a segment of the gastrointestinal tract. Each section is further divided into three parts: 1) the effects of wine on normal function; 2) the effects of wine in pathologic conditions; and 3) specific situations in which the use of wine is contraindicated. A special section at the beginning of the volume lists references which deal with the effects of wine on the digestive system in general, and includes a commentary on works whose pertinent text is cited in more than one of the subsections.

To enhance the value of this bibliography, each section is preceded by an introductory note explaining the function of that specific segment of the gastrointestinal tract and epitomizing the most important references to that segment. Furthermore, all pertinent references are annotated to indicate whether they are of interest as literature and history, or whether they bear scientific value. These latter are carefully collated and briefed. Limited quotations are used in order to give color and substance to the theme. References which are vague and of no particular interest are listed without comment for purposes of completeness. An author index, arranged alphabetically, is appended to aid the reader in his search for specific references.

In reviewing the data here presented, it becomes clear that although we of the scientific age belittle the use of home-remedies, nostrums, and other devices, some are worthy of our thoughtful concern especially in the light of the ultimate uses they serve in human history. As an illustration, the revival of interest in Indian snake-root *(Rauwolfia serpentina)* indicates the wisdom often concealed in empirical authority.

In our consideration of wine, the unbiased scientist and physician must admit that it is more than a beverage containing alcohol. There is no question but that it is capable of fulfilling certain human needs—psychologic as well as physiologic. As the literature here cited illustrates, wine, if properly used, stimulates appetite, excites gastrointestinal secretory functions, and is both a masterful and powerful therapeutic agent in a variety of disorders including many that involve the digestive system.

A field in which wine may be most sapiently used is geriatrics where its cardinal effect is euphorant; in addition, as part of the diet it furnishes vitamins and minerals as well as calories; when taken before a meal, it stimulates appetite and relieves tensions which might otherwise interfere with digestion; and when taken at bedtime, it gently beckons to Morpheus. Not only in geriatrics is wine worthy of our consideration, but it holds an equal place in the management of selected organic diseases. It is also a rich medicine in convalescence where it is indicated either as therapeutic agent or as adjuvant.

The ancient witch doctor made full use of exotic and rare ingredients—and these were usually offered in wine—the more to impress the patients. The modern physician, unwittingly follows the same pattern by excluding from his materia medica that which is always at hand and common knowledge. Whether wine be considered as food or medicine, whether ritualistically essential or religiously taboo, its 4,000-year-old history demonstrates effectively that it is the "most healthful of [dietary] beverages." (Pasteur).

SALVATORE P. LUCIA, M.D.

1   The Effects of Wine and its Constituents on the Overall Functions of the Gastrointestinal System

EFFECTS ON NORMAL FUNCTIONS

The gastrointestinal system is involved basically in the survival of the individual, since anything which is of value to the body, whatever its ultimate destination, is received and dispersed by some part of this system. Every imbibant or ingestant traverses the gastrointestinal tract where it is received, acted upon, and utilized or expelled. The reception of any food substance may be a psychophysiologic function, but its ultimate destiny concerns organophysiologic phenomena.

In the healthy human being, the work of the gastrointestinal tract begins with excitation of appetite before actual ingestion of the food. This is essential to the process of utilization of food. Following the ingestion of a food, digestion begins in the mouth and it is completed in the intestines. Each segment of the tract performs a specific function in this process.

The references in this section of the bibliography deal with the effects of wine—or some of its components—on digestion in general and are not specific to the function of any particular organ of the gastrointestinal tract.

The first physician to comment on wine as an aid to digestion—and the well-being of the individual in general—was Hippocrates. In the same vein followed Galen, and after him Celsus and the many other medical writers of the ensuing centuries. Most of the prescriptions of the master physicians were part of a total regimen designed to keep the individual well and fit; the specific value of wine to the gastrointestinal tract constituted only a passing reference. A good example of this type of commentary is the following quotation from a quaint book by Peter Shaw entitled *The Juice of the Grape*.

"Wine drunk in moderate quantities, or proportionably to the respective constitutions of men, in health, has a power to give sudden refreshment, to warm the stomach, gently stimulate its fibers, promote digestion, raise the pulse, rarify the blood, add to its velocity, open obstructions, forward excretions, greatly promote insensible perspiration, increase the natural strength, and enlarge the faculties of body and mind."

A fair appraisal of the evidence at hand would seem to indicate that wine does have a salutary effect on the healthy gastrointestinal tract both psychologically and physiologically. There is evidence for its being involved in initiating appetite as well as stimulating the digestive juices from the mouth to the intestines. By stimulating appetite as well as secretions, wine excites the digestive functions throughout. In large quantities, however, it tends to impede digestion by its depressant effect.

In general, the literature reporting the effect of wine on the gastrointestinal tract is still based mainly on clinical evaluation rather than on controlled experiment. The detailed consideration of wine as a dietary beverage indicates that its consumption paves the way for a better and more meaningful nutrition, since tensions and anxieties are thereby rendered less disturbing.

Fourth Century B.C.

Hippocrates HIPPOCRATES. WITH AN ENGLISH TRANSLATION BY W. H. S. JONES. *London: William Heinemann Ltd., New York: G. P. Putnam's Sons, 1923–1931, 4 vols. (The Loeb Classical Library)*

Although Hippocrates made extensive therapeutic use of wine, he did not elaborate on it in his writings. However, he did characterize wine as containing "something purgative from its original substance" and he did observe the retarding effects of wine on digestion. "Dark and harsh wines . . . pass well neither by stool nor by urine, nor by spittle." (Vol. IV, pp. 325–327) He also observed that the yeast and unaltered sugar of new wines are irritants of the gastrointestinal tract.

First Century A.D.

Celsus DE MEDICINA. WITH AN ENGLISH TRANSLATION BY W. G. SPENCER. *London: William Heinemann, Ltd., Cambridge: Harvard University Press, 1935–1938, 3 vols. (The Loeb Classical Library)*

This is one of the earliest books on medicine in which the author, although not a physician, epitomizes the practices of his time with regard to types of wine to be used in medicine. He also outlines the use of specific wines for different disease entities. ". . . when it [the stomach] does not retain food, . . . the most suitable drink is wine cold, . . . after the vomiting, anything light or not unsuitable for the stomach can be given; if even that is not retained, give a cupful of wine every hour until the stomach settles down . . . Another method to suppress the diarrhoea is to . . . eat about half a pound of bread soaked in undiluted wine;" (Vol. I, pp. 401–405; 441)

Dioscorides DE UNIVERSA MEDICINA, IN: THE GREEK HERBAL OF DIOSCORIDES. ILLUSTRATED BY A BYZANTINE, A.D.512. ENGLISHED BY JOHN GOODYER, A.D. 1655. EDITED AND FIRST PRINTED, A.D. 1933, BY ROBERT T. GUNTHER. *London: Oxford University Press, 1934.*

A compendium of medicinal wines written by a Greek army surgeon in the service of Nero. He has been called the founder of materia medica because he was the first to write on medical botany as an applied science. His precise descriptions of hundreds of substances, with their dietetic and therapeutic values appended, influenced physicians and pharmacists for 16 centuries. Dioscorides advised the use of wine, as had his Graeco-Roman predecessors, for countless ailments, always specifying a particular type. He noted the specific effects of old and new, dry and sweet wines on the nervous system, the digestive tract, the kidneys, and the urinary bladder.

Second Century A.D.

Galen OEUVRES ANATOMIQUES, PHYSIOLOGIQUES ET MEDICALES DE GALIEN. *Ch. Daremberg, translator. Paris: J. B. Baillière, 1854–1856, 2 vols.*

"If the stomach orifice is inflamed . . . and when this organ is weakened, one should give warm wine. If one cannot cause vomiting and relaxation of the stomach with warm water or a mixture of water and olive oil . . . one should give to drink an infusion of the heads of absinthia in melikraton [wine mixed with honey], then wine." (Vol. II, p. 736)

1478

Arnald of Villanova THE EARLIEST PRINTED BOOK ON WINE. NOW FOR THE FIRST TIME RENDERED INTO ENGLISH AND WITH AN HISTORICAL ESSAY BY HENRY E. SIGERIST, M.D. WITH FAC-SIMILE OF THE ORIGINAL EDITION, 1478. *New York: Schuman's, 1943.*

The earliest printed book on wine thought to be written in the thirteenth century by a person whose knowledge and objectivity brought the subject into proper focus. This is an important tract historically, philosophically, and practically. The observations are astute and remarkable for their time. Referable to the stomach, typical of his advice is the following:

"Raisin wine . . . strengthens the stomach, adds substance to the liver and strengthens it . . . And the wine made from fennel seeds . . . drives out flatulence and strengthens digestion . . . Wine made from anise . . . protects one from colic and flatulence and rectifies digestion and stops humid belching." (pp. 34, 39–40)

1493

The Kalendar & Compost of Shepherds FROM THE ORIGINAL EDITION PUBLISHED BY GUY MARCHANT IN PARIS IN THE YEAR 1493, AND TRANSLATED INTO ENGLISH C.1518; NEWLY EDITED FOR THE YEAR 1931, *by* G. C. HESELTINE. *London: Peter Davies, 1930.*

A volume of folkloric advice based on the four elements of Pythagoras. Written in the spirit of the doctrine of humors, it is a cyclical regimen organized loosely in zodiacal form. The program and regimen listed are in the character of a calendar with appended quaint essays. The volume is embellished with delightful wood blocks.

1568

Turner, William A BOOK OF WINES. TOGETHER WITH A MODERN ENGLISH VERSION OF THE TEXT BY THE EDITORS AND A GENERAL INTRODUCTION BY SANFORD V. LARKEY, M.D. AND AN OENOLOGICAL NOTE BY PHILIP M. WAGNER. *New York: Scholar's Facsimiles and Reprints, 1941.*

Written by a physician and botanist of the 16th century, this book is a treatise on the nature and properties of all wines commonly used in England at that time. As a physician, William Turner emphasizes the medical uses of wine and bases his recommendations mostly on the authority of the ancients, but occasionally cites from his own experience. As the subtitle explains, this book was intended as "a confutation of an error of some men, that hold, that Rhenish and and other small white wines ought not to be drunken of them that either have or are in danger of the stone, the rheum, and divers other diseases."

1586

Pisanelli, Baldassare TRATTATO DELLA NATURA DE'CIBI ET DEL BERE. NELQUALE NON SOLO TUTTE LE VIRTU, E I UITII DI QUELLI MINUTAMENTE SI PALESANO; MA ANCO I RIMEDII PER CORREGGERE I LORO DIFETTI COPIOSAMENTE S'INSEGNANO; TANTO NELL' APPARECCHIARLI PER L'USO QUANTO NELL'ORDINARE IL MODO DI RICEURERLI. *In Venetia, Appresso Gio. Alberti.*

A sixteenth century classic of a famous Bolognese physician in which the virtues of food and wine are given in great detail, and in which dosages of various wines are given to "maintain health." The book was first published in 1584 and was followed by many editions.

Although advising the moderate use of wine for all, the author denies it to children because it "adds fire unto the flames," and because it "disturbs the mind." (p. 136) "It [wine] increases and reawakens the appetite in the convalescent . . . it aids in the evacuation of excrements from the body." (pp. 137–138)

1638

Whitaker, Tobias THE TREE OF HUMANE LIFE, OR, THE BLOUD OF THE GRAPE, PROVING THE POSSIBILITIE OF MAINTAINING HUMANE LIFE FROM INFANCY TO EXTREAME OLD AGE WITHOUT ANY SICKNESSE BY THE USE OF WINE. *London: Printed by I. D. for H. O.*

An early and quaint treatise on the use of wine in medicine, based almost entirely on the teachings of Galen. It is primarily of historical value.

"Wine that is white, subtile and thinne, is not turbulent to the stomach, but is of easy digestion, soon penetrateth the veins." (p. 26)

1697

Lémery, Nicolas PHARMACOPEE UNIVERSELLE, CONTENANT TOUTES LES COMPOSITIONS DE PHARMACIE QUI SONT EN USAGE DANS LA MEDECINE . . . *Paris, L. d'Houry.*

A compilation of pharmaceutical recipes, apparently published at the expense of a drug house, with a section devoted to medicated wines. The author gives formulas and the mode of action for: Vinum Nephreticum Banderoni, Vinum Magistrale Purgans, Vinum Febrifugum, Vinum Martiale, Vinum Emeticum aut stibiatum, Vinum Hippocraticum, and Cerevitia purgativa D. Sydenham.

1705
Lémery, Louis TRAITE DES ALIMENTS . . . *Paris: P. Witte, Second edition. (First edition, J. B. Cusson et P. Witte, 1702)*

The tenor of this treatise is very aptly expressed in the following paragraph: "The good effects which wines produce, when taken moderately, provide mainly spiritual principles which aid digestion of aliments in the stomach, by communicating to this organ a gentle warmth . . . They give increased force to the blood; they affect the brain, giving beautiful thoughts and exciting memory. These spirits make all parts stronger and more vigorous." (p. 489)

1724
Shaw, P. THE JUICE OF THE GRAPE: OR, WINE PREFERABLE TO WATER. A TREATISE, WHEREIN WINE IS SHEWN TO BE THE GRAND PRESERVER OF HEALTH, AND RESTORER IN MOST DISEASES. WITH MANY INSTANCES OF CURES PERFORM'D BY THIS NOBLE REMEDY; AND THE METHOD OF USING IT, AS WELL AS FOR PREVENTION AS CURE. *By a fellow of the College. London: Printed for W. Lewis.*

An essay in which the medical virtues of wine are extolled. Most of the recommendations and conclusions are based on the author's personal observations and illustrated by case histories. "Wine drunk in moderate quantities, or proportionably to the respective constitutions of men, in health, has a power to give sudden refreshment, to warm the stomach, gently stimulate its fibers, promote digestion, raise the pulse, rarify the blood, add to its velocity, open obstructions, forward excretions, greatly promote insensible perspiration, increase the natural strength and the faculties of body and mind." (p.8)

1750
Graham, William THE ART OF MAKING WINES FROM FRUITS, FLOWERS, AND HERBS, ALL THE NATIVE GROWTH OF GREAT BRITAIN. PARTICULARLY OF GRAPES, GOOSEBERRIES, CURRANTS, RASBERRIES . . . WITH A SUCCINCT ACCOUNT OF THEIR MEDICINAL VIRTUES . . . *London: J. Williams.*

The medical advice is folkloric.

1787
Croft, John A TREATISE ON THE WINES OF PORTUGAL; AND WHAT
CAN BE GATHERED ON THE SUBJECT AND NATURE OF THE WINES,
&C., SINCE THE ESTABLISHMENT OF THE ENGLISH FACTORY AT
OPORTO, ANNO 1727: ALSO, A DISSERTATION ON THE NATURE AND
USE OF WINES IN GENERAL, IMPORTED INTO GREAT-BRITAIN, AS
PERTAINING TO LUXURY AND DIET. IN TWO PARTS. *New York:*
Crask and Lund.

A historical sketch on Port wines by a "member of the factory at Oporto, and wine-merchant, York" describing the development of the trade between England and Portugal. The
second part, on the "Nature and Use of Wines," gives the
characteristics and appropriate medical use of Rhenish wines,
Hungarian wines, French wines, Madeira wine, Canary wine,
Sherry wine, and Italian wines.

1795
Wright, John AN ESSAY ON WINES, ESPECIALLY ON PORT WINE;
INTENDED TO INSTRUCT EVERY PERSON TO DISTINGUISH THAT
WHICH IS PURE AND TO GUARD AGAINST THE FRAUDS OF ADUL-
TERATION; ALSO TO INDICATE WHEN AND HOW IT MAY BE USEFUL
OR INJURIOUS IN HEALTH OR DISEASE. *London: J. Barker.*

1799
Sandford, William A FEW PRACTICAL REMARKS ON THE MEDIC-
INAL EFFECTS OF WINE AND SPIRITS WITH OBSERVATIONS ON THE
OECONOMY OF HEALTH. INTENDED PRINCIPALLY FOR THE USE
OF PARENTS, GUARDIANS, AND OTHERS INTRUSTED WITH THE
CARE OF YOUTH. *Worcester: J. Tymbs.*

A delightful discursion on the medicinal effects of wine
and spirits containing quaint descriptions of physiologic effects. The author, surgeon to the Worcester Infirmary, states
in the preface that these "Practical Remarks [are] not as intended to prohibit altogether the *use* of wine or spirits, but
merely to discourage the very pernicious, and even fatal *abuse*
of them; . . ."

1815
Canu, F. RECHERCHES SUR L'HISTORIE, LA NATURE, LES EFFETS
DU VIN. *Paris: Thesis #270.*

A thesis written at the time when wine was to many the
panacea for all ills. "Wine acts as a tonic on the membranes
of the stomach; it exalts the vital properties . . . affected sym-

pathetically, all of the digestive organs which participate in
the stimulation of the stomach: liver, pancreas, salivary
glands . . ." (p.16)

1817
Loebenstein-Loebel, Ed. TRAITE SUR L'USAGE ET LES EFFETS
DES VINS DANS LES MALADIES DANGEREUSES ET MORTELLES ET
SUR LA FALSIFICATION DE CETTE BOISSON . . . *Translated from the
German by J. Fr. Daniel Lobstein. Strasbourg: F. G. Levrault.*

As stated in the title, a treatise on the use and effects of
wine. Written by a renowned French clinician, the detailed
recommendations including varieties of wine, amounts, and
recipes for medicated wines for specific diseases are based
on the author's clinical experience. Although the author discusses contraindications to the medicinal use of wine, the
supportive data offered fails in that it lacks discrimination.

1821
Baudot, L. A. ESSAI SUR L'EMPLOI HYGIENIQUE DU VIN. *Paris:
Thesis #178.*

In this essay wine is recommended for persons who have
painful, slow digestion, but contraindicated in the presence
of irritable digestion. The generalization is made that men
of letters suffer from constipation.

1824
Henderson, Alexander THE HISTORY OF ANCIENT AND MODERN
WINES. *London: Baldwin, Cradock, and Joy.*

A scholarly history of vineyards, vinification, and types of
wine in the ancient world as well as in modern Europe, Persia,
and Cape of Good Hope. The last chapter is devoted to the
dietetic and medical qualities of wine. Here the author, a
London physician, reviews the therapeutic use of wine by the
Greeks and Romans and gives his views on the advantages and
disadvantages of such usage. "Even in this light [when temperately used], it [wine] is to be viewed as a medicine rather than
as a beverage adapted to common use; . . . In general, then,
we may conclude, that the good effects of wine, as an article
of diet, are referable to its stimulating operation on the nervous and muscular coats of the stomach, by which means that
organ is incited to greater action and the flow of gastric juice
is promoted." (pp. 349–350)

Kitchiner, William THE ART OF INVIGORATING AND PROLONGING
LIFE BY FOOD, CLOTHES, AIR, EXERCISE, WINE, SLEEP, &c. AND

PEPTIC PRECEPTS, POINTING OUT AGREEABLE AND EFFECTUAL METHODS TO PREVENT AND RELIEVE INDIGESTION, AND TO REGULATE AND STRENGTHEN THE ACTION OF THE STOMACH AND BOWELS. *London: Hurst, Robinson, and Co., Fifth edition. (First edition, c. 1821)*

The author discusses wine as one of the elements of longevity. Amounts are given for the most beneficial use of wine. Included is such unusual advice as: "Feeble persons, who are subject to such sudden attacks [of exhaustion] should always travel armed with a *Pocket Pistol* charged with a couple of glasses of White Wine, . . ." (p. 200)

1826
Gardeton, C. G. DICTIONNAIRE DES ALIMENS. PRECEDE D'UNE HYGIENE DES TEMPERAMENS, DE REFLEXIONS SUR LA DIGESTION ET LES MALADIES DE L'ESTOMAC, ETC. *Paris: J. J. Naudin.*

Written by a physician, the actual "Dictionary" is preceded by a discussion of temperaments, digestion, and diseases of the stomach. The "Dictionary" gives accurate descriptions of the medicinal wines in use at that time (about 17 formulas) with discussions for their use, as well as directions for the use of "ardent and spirituous liquors."

1827
Bonguiod, D. CONSIDERATIONS SUR LES QUALITES ET L'USAGE DU VIN. *Paris: Thesis #191.*

A thesis in general terms on the qualities of wine and its uses in health and disease. The advice given is not specific; it emphasizes "wise" use and enumerates contraindications. With reference to the digestive system, the author states: "Administered wisely, it sustains the stomach, and the whole organism feels its good effects; but this liquor so salutary for some, is a fatal poison for others; the greatest temperance should direct its use." (p. 9)

1831
Beaurepaire, L. B. DISSERTATION SUR LE VIN. *Paris: Thesis #155.*

A dissertation dealing with the uses of wine in nutritional deficiencies, chronic and infectious diseases, diseases of the gastrointestinal tract, genito-urinary tract, and of the nervous system and in mental diseases. The main theme, however, seems to be that "wine is all-powerful in sustaining the principle of life." (p. 16)

Stuart, Moses AN ESSAY UPON THE WINES AND STRONG DRINKS OF THE ANCIENT HEBREWS, AND THEIR REFERENCE TO DIETETIC AND RELIGIOUS VIEWS ON THE MODERN USE OF SPIRITUOUS LIQUORS, BEING AN ANSWER TO THE QUESTION, WHETHER THE USE OF DISTILLED LIQUORS OR TRAFFIC IN THEM, IS COMPATIBLE, AT THE PRESENT TIME, WITH MAKING A PROFESSION OF CHRISTIANITY . . . *Reprinted from the American edition. With a preface by John Pye Smith. London: E. Wilson.*

An essay in which the drinking habits of the ancient Hebrews, as recorded in the Bible and other works on the subject, are analyzed and the conclusion is drawn that "an injunction to drink a little pure wine, the simple juice of the grape, is not a permission to drink a great deal of wine, flaming with alcohol . . ." (p. 15)

1839
Aulagnier, A. F. DICTIONNAIRE DES ALIMENS ET LES BOISSONS EN USAGE DANS LES DIVERS CLIMATS ET CHEZ LES DIFFERENS PEUPLES . . . PRECEDE DE CONSIDERATIONS GENERALES SUR LA NOURRITURE DE L'HOMME . . . *Paris: Cousin.*

In his discussion on wines, the author states: "Heavy wines are very nourishing; the old are tonic, and suitable for weak stomachs. Fine wines are less nourishing than others, but are more easily digested." (p. 706)

The author also classifies wines according to their origin and discusses their medicinal values. "Wines of Rhaetia are stomachics . . . The wine of Alicante, when not falsified, is both stomachic and tonic." (pp. 710, 719)

1841–1845
Lévy, Michel TRAITE D'HYGIENE PUBLIQUE ET PRIVEE. *Paris: J. B. Baillière et fils, 2 vols.*

In the first volume of this work the author, a professor of medicine, discusses the influence of such varied agents as temperament, age, sex, heredity, customs, environment (natural and artificial) on individual hygiene; in the second volume he discusses solid foods, beverages, clothing, exercise, and lastly public hygiene. In his elaboration on foods, one chapter is devoted to alcoholic beverages both fermented and distilled.

1851
Carpenter, William B. ON THE USE AND ABUSE OF ALCOHOLIC LIQUORS IN HEALTH AND DISEASE. PRIZE ESSAY. *London: Charles*

Gilpin & John Churchill.

Written as an essay for a contest sponsored by Drs. Forbes (Physician to the Household of Queen Victoria), Roupell and Guy, it was awarded the first prize and published in book form in 1849; it was re-issued in 1851.

The author is of the opinion that the temperance movement will fail because of human frailty; that what is needed is a "Total Abstinence Movement." He discusses at length the effect of alcohol on the body and mental powers, and poses the question: is alcohol a necessary medicine?

With regard to the digestive system, the author considers alcohol to act in two ways: ". . . first, by the direct irritating action of the fluid upon the mucous lining of the Alimentary Canal; and second, by the general deterioration of the nutritive processes, resulting in various ways from the entrance of Alcohol into the Blood . . . A small quantity of alcoholic liquor, diluted by the fluids already in the stomach, appears to produce only the first effect, namely, a quickening of the circulation, and a temporary exaltation of the functional activity of the organ, as shown in the increase of appetite and of digestive power . . . Where, in place of excessive indulgence, what is commonly considered a *moderate* use has been made of Alcoholic liquors, we cannot with the same confidence attribute to it any decided departure from the healthy condition of the Stomach; and it is certain that the mucous membrane becomes in time so habituated to its presence, that its contact no longer produces the same effects as it does on a membrane unaccustomed to it." (pp. 51–52; 59)

1852

McMullen, Thomas HANDBOOK OF WINES, PRACTICAL, THEORETICAL, AND HISTORICAL; WITH A DESCRIPTION OF FOREIGN SPIRITS AND LIQUEURS. *New York: D. Appleton and Company.*

A text compiled to provide "authentic information upon the subject of Wines," it discusses: grapes and grapevines; fermentation, vinification and vintage; the wines of Europe, Persia and Cape of Good Hope; storing, mixing and adulteration of wines; the dietetic and medical qualities of wines; alcoholic strength of wines; and, liqueurs. The volume has two appendices, one listing wines and their geographical origin, the other listing alcoholic liquors and their geographical origin. The chapter on the dietetic and medicinal value of wine is presented by Dr. Alexander Henderson. (see pp. 199–215)

1857
Gaubert, P. ETUDE SUR LES VINS ER LES CONSERVES, SUIVIE DU COMPTE RENDU DE LA SEANCE DE DEGUSTATION TENUE PAR LES MEMBRES DE LA IIE CLASSE DE L'EXPOSITION UNIVERSELLE. *Paris: Mme Croissant.*

"In general, wines in small quantity, when taken at any stage of a meal, facilitate and accelerate digestion . . . The acidity of some white wines, however, may irritate the stomach and thus hinder digestion rather than aid it. It is in the intelligent diluting that white wine appears destined to render great service." (pp. 128, 161)

1862
Tovey, Charles WINE AND WINE COUNTRIES. A RECORD AND MANUAL FOR WINE MERCHANTS AND WINE CONSUMERS. *London: Hamilton, Adams & Co.*

This book, aside from describing the various wines, draws attention to some of the frauds perpetrated in the wine trade and alerts the consumer to such fraudulent practices. The book discusses wine consumption in England, the wines of Europe, America, and the British colonies, and the chemistry and medicinal value of wine. In the chapter on wine as a medicine, the author states that Hippocrates preferred it as a generous cordial. (p. 285) The author further quotes from Dr. Henderson who felt that, when temperately used, wine acts as a stimulant quickening the heart and arteries, and promoting the different secretions. (p. 286) Hock is advised for the treatment of obesity. (p. 297)

1864
Denman, James L. THE VINE AND ITS FRUIT. MORE ESPECIALLY IN RELATION TO THE PRODUCTION OF WINE: EMBRACING AN HISTORICAL AND DESCRIPTIVE ACCOUNT OF THE GRAPE, ITS CULTURE AND TREATMENT IN ALL COUNTRIES, ANCIENT AND MODERN. DRAWN FROM THE BEST AUTHORITIES, AND INCORPORATING A BRIEF DISCOURSE ON WINE. *London: Longman, Green, Longman, Roberts, & Green.*

A revision and extension of the original pamphlet entitled "A Brief Discourse on Wine," replete with scholarly details and quotations and interlaced with medical advice and recommendations all based on ancient and contemporary medical writings.

1865
Druitt, Robert REPORT ON THE CHEAP WINES OF FRANCE, ITALY,

AUSTRIA, GREECE, AND HUNGARY; THEIR QUALITY, WHOLESOME-
NESS, AND PRICE, AND THEIR USE IN DIET AND MEDICINE. WITH
SHORT NOTES OF A LECTURE TO LADIES ON WINE, AND REMARKS
ON ACIDITY. *London: Henry Renshaw.*

Written after Gladstone lowered the import duties on wine,
it is a defense of these "cheap" wines, describing them and
giving their various uses. This work was intended primarily
for the medical practitioner—to familiarize him with the
characteristics of the various wines and thus enable him to
use them most profitably in his practice. The author's recommendations of wine are based principally on his own experience as a clinician and officer of health. "In prescribing *wine,*
the judicious practitioner desires to give not merely *alcohol,*
but a liquid containing the saline and extractive parts of grape-
juice, . . . those powerful oils and ethers which give wine its
bouquet and its marvellous exhilarating properties. True *wine,*
as has been well said, contains more mineral ingredients than
many a mineral water." (p. 22) A second edition, "rewritten
and enlarged," appeared in 1873.

1868
Beckwith, Edward Lonsdale PRACTICAL NOTES ON WINE. *London: Smith, Elder and Co.*

The author, juror and reporter on the wines at the Paris
Exhibition of 1867, gives his unscientific opinion on the physiologic effects of wine.

c. 1873
Bégin, E. EMPLOI DU VIN DE BAGNOLS (ST. RAPHAEL) DANS
LES HOPITAUX DE PARIS. *Paris: J. B. Baillière et fils.*

1876
Blanchin, X. LE VIN DE SAINT-RAPHAEL NATUREL, COMPARE
AUX VINS PHARMACEUTIQUES. *Gaz. Hôp. 49:1156.*

1877
Anstie, Frances E. ON THE USES OF WINES IN HEALTH AND DIS-
EASE. *London: Macmillan and Co.*

A two-part monograph which first appeared in the *Practitioner.* Part I deals with the place of wine in the daily diet
and Part II with the uses of wines in acute and chronic diseases. The author bases his opinions on his personal clinical
experience and observations; he gives doses and dosages for
various wines and medicated wines in the different illnesses.

Bégin, E. WINE IN THE DIFFERENT FORMS OF ANAEMIA AND ATONIC GOUT. *(Translated from the French) Paris: J. B. Baillière et fils.*

"Astringent and sweet tannic wines, such as Saint Raphaël, far surpass in a hygienic point of view, those which are simply alcoholic or alcoholic and sweet, because they agree better with the digestive organs when they are taken in moderate doses." (p. 8)

Husson, C. DU VIN, SES PROPRIETES, SA COMPOSITION, SA PREPARATION, SES MALADIES ET LES MOYENS DE LES GUERIR, SES FALSIFICATIONS ET LES PROCEDES USITES POUR LES RECONNAITRE. *Paris: P. Asselin.*

An essay in which the author upholds the theme that the liquorous wines are useful for "cold stomachs and are good to dissipate the heaviest of the stomach caused by raw and undigested matter." (p. 49)

The author is of the opinion that in contagious dysentery, when the skin is cold, the face wrinkled, the pulse threadlike and there is considerable prostration, wine is indicated.

1886

Roberts, Sir William LECTURES ON DIETETICS AND DYSPEPSIA. DELIVERED AT THE OWENS COLLEGE SCHOOL OF MEDICINE IN FEBRUARY AND MARCH 1885. *London: Smith, Elder & Co., Second edition. (First edition, 1885)*

Five lectures discussing dietetics in general, effect of food-accessories on salivary digestion, on peptic digestion, on pancreatic digestion, and on the acid dyspepsia of healthy persons.

Rochard, J. L'ALCOOL—SON ROLE DANS LES SOCIETES MODERNES. *Rev. Deux Mondes, 74:871–900.*

The author recommends wine as the most beneficent of all alcoholic beverages. He describes it as a happy combination of alcohol, tannin and aroma: "Of all beverages, the best known and most inoffensive is *wine*. All its elements happily combined produce lazier digestion and slower absorption; they lessen the effects of alcohol on the stomach and moderate its action on the nervous system." (p. 873)

1887

Gustafson, Axel THE FOUNDATION OF DEATH: A STUDY OF THE DRINK QUESTION. *New York: Funk & Wagnalls, Third edition. (First edition, 1884)*

A defense of the prohibitionist point of view. The author, although biased, presents a vast amount of information—historical, medical, and social. The topics covered are: Drinking among the ancients; history of the discovery of distillation; preliminaries to the study of modern drinking; universality of liquor adulteration; effects of alcohol on the physical organs and functions; diseases caused by alcohol; moral results of drinking; effects of alcohol on heredity; alcohol as a medicine; the general effects of alcohol on society; origin and causes of alcoholism; specious reasonings concerning the use of alcohol; and the temperance movement. Appended to the book is a bibliography of some 560 items.

In the two chapters dealing with the physiologic effects and therapeutic use of alcohol, the author quotes such medical authorities as Drs. Carpenter, Flint, Lee, Beaumont, and others.

1898
Chittenden, R. H., L. B. Mendel, and H. C. Jackson A FURTHER STUDY OF THE INFLUENCE OF ALCOHOL AND ALCOHOLIC DRINKS UPON DIGESTION, WITH SPECIAL REFERENCE TO SECRETION. *Amer. J. Physiol., 1:164–209.*

One of the earliest experimental studies in which the influence of alcohol and various alcoholic beverages upon digestion are compared. In this study, the authors are concerned mainly with the action of alcoholic beverages on secretion. Their findings report on: salivary secretion; the influence of alcoholic fluids in the mouth; on gastric secretion and gastric digestion. The beverages used were: whiskey, sherry, white wine, claret, beer, porter, and water. Both animal (dogs) and human subjects were used.

1900
Allen, Martha M. ALCOHOL. A DANGEROUS AND UNNECESSARY MEDICINE. HOW AND WHY. WHAT MEDICAL WRITERS SAY. *Marcellus (New York): Department of Medical Temperance of the National Woman's Christian Temperance Union.*

Written by the Superintendent of the Department of Medical Temperance for the National Woman's Christian Temperance Union, the book treats alcohol in that perspective; it epitomizes the history of alcohol, of the temperance movement and gives a listing of temperance hospitals. The book is replete with selected and prejudiced quotations from physicians and other scientists.

1902

Cayla, F. ALIMENTS, BOISSONS ET CONDIMENTS. REPAS DES ADULTES ET DES VIEILLARDS SAINS, VALETUDINAIRES OU MALADES. *Paris and Bordeaux: Vigot frères and G. Gounouilhou.*

A handbook on nutrition, written by the retired chairman of the then medical clinic of Bordeaux, and presenting the characteristic prejudices of the locality. The book covers caloric and nutritional value of various foods and beverages; in discussing spices, Professor Cayla likens their physiologic effect to that of alcohol. One section is devoted to the diet in dyspepsia, convalescence, and in some other conditions. To the book is appended an essay contrasting wine and the wine-drinker with the drinker of distilled spirits.

Lusk, Graham THE COMMON USE OF ALCOHOL AS A BEVERAGE. *Boston Med. Surg. J., 147:43–45.*

A paper first read at the meeting of the Massachusetts Medical Society, discussing the subject in very general terms. "On the whole, the moderate use of alcohol as a beverage gives additional flavor to the food, and acts as a mild narcotic, often preceded by a period of exhilaration." (p. 45).

Russillet, Maurice: LE VIN. *Lyon: Thesis #29.*

1903

Billings, John S. PHYSIOLOGICAL ASPECTS OF THE LIQUOR PROBLEM. *Boston and New York: Houghton, Mifflin and Company, 2 vols.*

A collection of several reports on the various aspects of the Liquor Problem, begun in 1897 under the auspices of the Committee of Fifty. The investigations reported in these volumes were carried out under the direction of W. O. Atwater, John S. Billings, H. P. Bowditch, R. H. Chittenden, and W. H. Welch. Volume I includes reports on: The Present Instruction on the Physiological Action of Alcohol, by H. P. Bowditch and C. F. Hodge; The Influence of Alcohol and Alcoholic Beverages on Digestion and Secretion, by R. H. Chittenden; Data Relating to the Use of Alcoholic Drinks among Brain Workers in the United States, by J. S. Billings; Relations of Drink Habits to Insanity, by J. S. Billings; The Influence of Alcohol on Growth and Development, by C. F. Hodge; The Influence of Acute Alcoholism on the Normal Vital Resistance of Rabbits to Infection, by A. C. Abbott.

Volume II includes: A Critical Review of the Pharmacological Action of Ethyl Alcohol, with A Statement of the Relative Toxicity of the Constituents of Alcoholic Beverages, by John J. Abel; The Nutritive Value of Alcohol, by W. O. Atwater; The Use of "Temperance Drinks," by H. P. Bowditch; and, The Pathological Effects of Alcohol, by William H. Welch. Experiments, as well as descriptive studies on both man and animals and on natural and artificial digestion, are reported.

Mauriac, E. LE VIN AU POINT DE VUE MEDICAL, SA COMPOSITION CHIMIQUE, SES PROPRIETES THERAPEUTIQUES, SES INDICATIONS ET SES CONTREINDICATIONS DANS LE TRAITEMENT DES MALADIES. *Paris: O. Doin.*

As a clinician, the author discusses the various French wines and their suitability in specific diseases. "In our opinion, the red wines would always occupy the first position, not only from the alimentary point of view, but also from the therapeutic point of view. They are powerful tonics and adjuvants, without being stimulating or fatiguing to the stomach." (p. 12)

1907

Cayla, F. REGIMES PATHOLOGIQUES ET REGIME PARFAIT. *Paris: Vigot frères.*

For the everyday diet of the healthy adult, the author recommends "maximum 2 glasses of red or light white Bordeaux mixed with water, with the meal; in the summer, white Bordeaux mixed with carbonated water . . ." (p. 65)

Mauriac, E. LES VINS DE BORDEAUX, LEURS QUALITES HYGIENIQUES ET CURATIVES. *Bordeaux: Féret et fils.*

1909

Horsley, Sir Victor, and Mary D. Sturge ALCOHOL AND THE HUMAN BODY. AN INTRODUCTION TO THE STUDY OF THE SUBJECT, AND A CONTRIBUTION TO NATIONAL HEALTH. *London: Macmillan and Co., Limited. (First edition, 1907; Second edition, 1908; Special edition, April 1909, reprinted in June 1909.)*

A supporter of the British Temperance Union, the author, by reviewing experimental work done by others and relating his own observations, attempts to prove that alcohol is harmful to the healthy and unnecessary in medicine. Sir Victor discusses the chemistry of alcohol and alcoholic beverages; the effects of alcoholic beverages on the human organism in health and disease; and, the effects of alcohol on race and national health.

Pons, C., and Broeckaert SUR LA VALEUR ALIMENTAIRE DE L'AL-COOL. *Belgique Méd., 16:231–234.*

"Alcohol in small doses, such as in wine or beer, exercises stimulating effect on the gastric mucosa and the secretions of the stomach, salivary glands and pancreas . . . [It also] exerts a favorable influence on the motility of the stomach . . . the fats, for example, are more easily accepted and digested." (pp. 231–232)

Yorke-Davies, N. E. WINE AND HEALTH. HOW TO ENJOY BOTH. *London: Chatto & Windus.*

Written by a physician for lay readers, this book answers many questions which a layman might ask of his doctor. The book is divided into two parts. Part I discusses: the necessity and virtue of alcohol; is alcohol a food? is pure wine harmless? what wines to drink; foreign and English spirits; malt liquors, cider and perry; the worship of Bacchus; and, the excessive use of alcohol. Part II is concerned with diseases induced or influenced by alcohol: obesity, gout, rheumatism, indigestion, nervous ailments, Bright's disease, constipation, acidity, diabetes, and anemia. The author quotes extensively from the works of Drs. Parkes, Pavy, Hutchison, and other authorities, as well as from his own clinical experience.

1912

Fitch, W. E. THE FOOD AND MEDICINAL VALUE OF WINE. *Pediatrics, 24:102–108.*

In this article the value of wine as a food and medicine is reviewed. The author elaborates on the ideas of Atwater and Benedict, von Liebig, Crouzel, Duclaux, Mauriac, Pick, Sabrazès, and Mercadier, and concludes with the statement that "a dry brown tongue, restlessness and a feeble irregular pulse are the indications for the administration [of wine]."

1915

Brunet, Raymond LA VALEUR ALIMENTAIRE ET HYGIENIQUE DU VIN. *Paris: Librairie Agricole de la Maison Rustique, Fourth edition. (First edition, 1914)*

Brunet, owner of a vineyard and editor of the *Revue de Viticulture,* frankly states that the book was written in order to defend wine against accusations from any .quarter. He quotes medical authority on the physiologic and beneficial effects of wine. His defense is pertinently documented.

1916
Koren, John ALCOHOL AND SOCIETY. *New York: Henry Holt and Company.*

The author, an investigator of the Committee of Fifty, has assembled factual data on alcohol and presents the arguments concerning prohibition in an orderly and authoritative fashion. The volume is divided into five sections, as follows: I. Social Aspects of Drink. II. Drink Reform in the United States. II. Government and Prohibition. IV. Drink Reform in Foreign Countries. V. Constructive Temperance Reform.

1919
Flint, G. E. THE WHOLE TRUTH ABOUT ALCOHOL. *New York: Macmillan and Company.*

"The moderate drinking of wine, at meals is a valuable aid to digestion, not only because of the alcohol, but also owing to the water." (p. 153)

Rosewater, C. A. ALCOHOL AS A MEDICINE. ABSTRACTS FROM THE WRITINGS OF EMINENT AUTHORITIES. *J. Med. Soc. N.J., 16:274–282.*

A lecture presented at the annual meeting of the Medical Society of New Jersey, this article presents in abstract form the findings of: Drs. Abraham Jacobi, William Osler, William Edward Fitch, Charles Gilmore Kerley, L. Emmett Holt, Arthur R. Cushny, George Frederick Still, Chalmers Watson, Robert Hutchison, William Tibbles, Hobart Amory Hare, A. A. Brill, Charles E. de M. Sajous, Harvey W. Wiley, George F. Butler, H. Edward Lewis, Paul Bartholow, John William Springthrope, Samuel O. L. Potter, John V. Shoemaker, John H. Musser, W. Gilman Thompson, and Norman Kerr.

1920
Dale, H. H. DISCUSSION OF THE VALUE OF ALCOHOL AS A THERAPEUTIC AGENT. *Roy. Soc. Med. Proc. (Sect. Ther. & Pharmacol.), 13:31–58.*

A discussion by various participants on the pharmacologic value of alcohol as a therapeutic agent. Dr. Dale reviews the physiological and pharmacological evidence as to the actions of alcohol which can be experimentally demonstrated.

1923
Starling, Ernest H. THE ACTION OF ALCOHOL ON MAN, WITH ESSAYS ON: 1. ALCOHOL AS A MEDICINE, BY ROBERT HUTCHISON; 2. ALCOHOL AND ITS RELATION TO PROBLEMS IN MENTAL DISORDERS, BY SIR FREDERICK W. MOTT; 3. ALCOHOL AND MORALITY, BY RAYMOND PEARL. *London: Longmans, Green and Co.*

The book is divided into two parts. The first presents material on: fermentation and fermented liquors; the fate of alcohol in the body; foods, drugs, and poisons; alcohol as a food; action of alcohol on human behavior; effects of alcohol on fatigue; influence of alcohol on digestion; effects of alcohol on circulation of the blood; influence of alcohol on respiration and body temperature; effects of immoderate use of alcohol and its influence on the community. The second part of the book is an appendix consisting of the three essays named on the title page.

1927
Feldman, W. M. ALCOHOL IN ANCIENT JEWISH LITERATURE. *Brit. J. Inebriety 24:122–124.*

A sociologic discussion concerning the free use of wine in Jewish culture, where alcoholism is relatively unknown. In explanation, the following is advanced: (1) the use of alcohol within the family unit—as a food, a medicine, and as part of the religious ritual; and (2), respect for the Talmudic injunction that "wine should be taken only with meals; in between meals it intoxicates."

1928
Brooks, H. USE OF ALCOHOL IN THE CIRCULATORY DEFECTS OF OLD AGE. *Med. J. Rec., 127:199–201.*

A lecture presented before the Medical Association of Greater New York, which stresses the value of alcoholic beverages, particularly wine and beer, in the circulatory diseases of old age. "A glass of wine with meals . . . is a very satisfactory means of aiding digestion and increasing the caloric intake." (p. 200)

This paper is followed by a discerning discussion concerning the medicinal use of dietary beverage alcohol.

1929
Alquier, J. VALEUR BIOLOGIQUE ET HYGIENIQUE DU VIN. *Bull. Soc. Sci. Hyg. Aliment., 17:115–182.*

A survey of experimental work on man and animals relative to the physiological and psychological effects of wine. Included is a discussion of the importance of wine in the diet of the French people.

Crum, E. L. USE OF WINE IN ROMAN MEDICINE ACCORDING TO CELSUS. *Mich. State Med. Soc. J. 28:298–306.*

The author, a classicist, reviews the medical uses of wine by the early Romans and Greeks from materials available in the literature, particularly of Celsus and Pliny.

Loeper, M., and J. Alquier L'ACTION PHYSIOLOGIQUE ET THERAPEUTIQUE DU VIN. *Prog. Méd., 44:1725–1730.*

A combined report of experimental work on human and animal subjects, as well as clinical observations on the physiologic effect of wine as a therapeutic agent. "Our research confirms that wine in moderation excites digestion." (p. 1725)

1930

Delaunay, H., and G. Portmann DEFENSE MEDICALE ET PHYSIOLOGIQUE DU VIN. *Bull. Int. Vin, 3:50–64.*

"Wine stimulates digestive secretions . . . Prof. Pachon estimates that the most important action of wine is its psychic stimulating effect on the digestive secretions. From the physiologic point of view, the qualities of good wine—bouquet, aroma—act on the sense organs of sight, taste, smell. They modify favorably the psychic tonus, but this is only an accessory action. The principal action is the automatic releasing, by reflex, of gastric secretion." (pp. 55–56)

Renaud, M. VIN ET ALIMENTATION. *Rev. Crit. Path. Thérap. 1:315–320.*

The author recounts in characteristic French fashion the subjective response that "wine favors the organic functions of the gastrointestinal tract." (p. 318)

1931

Llaguet VIN EN HYGIENE ET EN MEDECINE. *J. Med. Bordeaux, 108:1065–1067.*

The virtues of wine as a therapeutic agent are heralded by a sympathetic physician and oenophile.

Pousson; Viennet, and J. Blanc VERITE SUR LE VIN *Bull. Int. Vin., 4:28–37.*

An article in which the "truth on wine" is presented in the form of an indiscriminate "praise of wine" as an antidote to alcoholism, an antiseptic, tonic, and elixir of longevity. Wine is recommended for all illnesses and all ages.

1932
Cuvier, F. LE VIN. *Paris: Thesis #200.*

A thesis in the usual form epitomizing past medical lore of wine with added benefit of new experimental verification. Characteristic of its content is the following: "Champagne calms and lulls the mucosa of the stomach. It is indicated in vomiting . . . The dry white wines . . . are suitable in hyperchlorhydria, dyspepsia, pyrosis, gastric pain." (p. 75) The author gives an account of an unusual experiment illustrating the effects and results of toxicity of breakdown products of beef, chicken, and rabbit when given to guinea pigs parenterally with and without concomitance of wine of St. Emilion.

1933
Allen, H. Warner SHERRY. WITH AN APPENDIX ON SHIPPERS AND A FOLDING MAP. *London: Constable & Co. Ltd.*

An eloquent description of Jerez and the making of sherry. On p. 97 will be found the author's credo: "A glass of sherry could certainly be good for patients, as it awakes the appetite and arouses the digestive juices."

Eylaud, J. M. VIN DE SAUTERNES ET LES MEDECINS. *Bull. Int. Vin.* 6:117–120.

A discussion of the beneficial physiologic effects of wine and some of its constituents—tannin, glycerides, minerals, acids, ethers—on the human body by one of the foremost exponents of the use of wine in medicine.

Eylaud, J. M., and R. Marcard VIN AU POINT DE VUE HYGIENIQUE. *Bull. Int. Vin,* 6:90–99.

The authors believe that wine used as an appetizer or digestive agent contributes "in the fight against alcoholism." The Sauternes, liqueurous wines with perceptible higher sugar and alcohol content, are considered "excitant tonics." The wines of Champagne are recommended in instances of vomiting or in "high fevers having need of a light wine which does not fatigue the stomach." (p. 94)

Stoll, Horatio F. WINE-WISE. *San Francisco*: *H. S. Crocker Press.*
"Sparkling wines are renowned as aids to digestion." (p. 53)

1934

Buytendijk, M. LES BIENFAITS SPECIFIQUES DU VIN. *IIe Congrès Nat'l. Méd. Amis des Vins de France, Béziers, pp. 304–317.*

An article in which the importance of the olfactory sense is discussed. The author is of the opinion that taste and smell are important to the total well-being of the adult, although this is a difficult proposition to prove by laboratory techniques. With this in mind, the author agrees with Professor Lagrange who considers wine to be "a tonic. It is indispensable to man and to prohibit it would be condemning humanity to a search for an unknown equivalent and thereby courting failure." (p. 304)

Dontas, S. LE VIN EN GRECE. UN VIN PARTICULIER. LE VIN COMME ALIMENT. OENISME ET ALCOOLISME. L'EXPERIENCE GRECQUE. *IIe Congrès Nat'l. Méd. Amis des Vins de France, Béziers, pp. 236–271.*

A rambling review of ancient medicinal uses of wine in Greece, with references modern and classical.

Fiessinger, Charles L'HYGIENE DES GENS PRESSES. TOME I. LA PRESERVATION DES MALADIES. *Paris: L'Etoile.*

A compilation of dietary regimens for the harrassed and overworked, in which the function of French wines is described.

Parcé LA VALEUR MEDECINALE DU VIN DE BANYULS. *IIe Congrès Nat'l. Méd. Amis des Vins de France, Béziers, pp. 69–75.*

1935

Dougnac, F. LE VIN, AUX POINTS DE VUE PHYSICO-CHIMIQUE, PHYSIOLOGIQUE, HYGIENIQUE, ET THERAPEUTIQUE. *Preface by Prof. Portmann. Bordeaux: Editions Delmas.*

An extensive review of experimental and clinical data relating to the physiochemical and physiological effects of wine, including its dietary value, and the use of wine in modern therapy. Although containing some unsupported statements, the book has value as an historical review of researches in the field of alcohol and its beverages.

1936

Bethea, O. W. THERAPEUTIC USE OF ALCOHOLIC BEVERAGES. *Int. Med. Dig., 28:369–373.*

A compilation of "recent expressions of leading pharmacologists" on the topic of the therapeutic use of alcoholic beverages. The article consists entirely of quotes out of context and is therefore difficult to evaluate.

Boulet, P. LE VIN CHAUD. *IIIe Congrès Nat'l. Méd. Amis des Vins de France, Dijon, pp. 41–44.*

An article in which the author, former mayor and deputy of the eminent wine community of Montpellier, discusses the advantages of giving soldiers mulled wine. Mulled wine, he states, is antiseptic, nutritive, tonic, stimulant, diaphoretic, and warming.

Derys, Gaston MON DOCTEUR LE VIN. AQUARELLES DE RAOUL DUFY. *Paris: Draeger Frères.*

The text consists entirely of quotes from famous physicians and delicate anecdotes accompanied by fine watercolor illustrations executed by Raoul Dufy.

des Ouches, M. LA THERAPEUTIQUE PAR LE VIN ET LES VINS MEDICINAUX. *IIIe Congrès Nat'l. Méd. Amis des Vins de France, Dijon, pp. 11–14.*

A eulogy to wine with recommendations for its use and a discussion of medicinal wines listed in the current French Pharmacopoeia.

Mistal, O. M. LE VIN EST-IL NUISIBLE AUX TUBERCULEUX? *IIIe Congrès Nat'l. Méd. Amis des Vins de France, Dijon, pp. 87–94.*

A review by a Swiss physician on the pro's and con's of the use of wine in tuberculosis. His conclusion, based on personal observation and on reported literature, is that moderate doses of wine are useful therapeutic aids in certain cases. "Agreeable to take, wine stimulates the appetite, facilitates digestion and assimilation of food, provokes a certain euphoria, exerts a favorable influence on the psychic state of the patient, and banishes fear." (p. 90)

1938

Jager, J. LA VALEUR ALIMENTAIRE ET THERAPEUTIQUE DU VIN. *Paris: Thesis #550. Also in Médecine, 19:990–993.*

"Wine taken in moderation is a food and a useful medicine for combatting a number of infections." (p. 993)

Marescalchi, A. L'AZIONE FISIOLOGICA DEL VINO SULLO STOMACO UMANO. *L'Italia Vinicola ed Agraria, 28:313–314.*

A review article in which "authorities" are cited who believe that wine has a beneficial effect on digestion.

1939
Guillermin, R. LES VINS EN THERAPEUTIQUE. *Praxis, 28:372–373.*

"Wine facilitates digestion, and assures better utilization of the ingested food . . . [it] is indicated in anorexia . . ."

Soula, G. LES PROPRIETES PHYSIOLOGIQUES ET PHARMACODYNAMIQUES DU VIN. *Conf. d'Oenologie Fac. Méd. Toulouse, pp. 32–35.*

A brief review of the physiologic and pharmacodynamic properties of wine presented at a conference of the Medical Faculty of Toulouse. With regard to the digestive system, the author, a professor of physiology, states that although experiments have shown that the action of digestive enzymes is not altered by moderate amounts of wine, the general effect of wine on digestion needs further investigation before any conclusions are drawn.

1940
Beazell, J. M., and A. C. Ivy THE INFLUENCE OF ALCOHOL ON THE DIGESTIVE TRACT. *Quart. J. Stud. Alc., 1:45–73.*

A review of the available scientific data on the effect of alcohol on various divisions of the gastrointestinal tract, as follows: the salivary glands, mouth and esophagus; gastric secretion; effect of habitual use of alcohol on the stomach; gastric motility; effect of alcohol on pancreatic secretion; alcoholism and pancreatitis; effect of alcohol on digestive enzymes and gastric digestion; absorption of alcohol; effect of alcohol on function of the liver; cirrhosis of the liver. The authors present their conclusions in a summary of the article. The conclusions on the various topics will be found in the appropriate subsections of this bibliography.

Jellinek, E. M., and N. Jolliffe EFFECTS OF ALCOHOL ON THE INDIVIDUAL. A REVIEW OF THE LITERATURE. *Quart. J. Stud. Alc., 1:110–181.*

A review of the literature published in the United States and Europe during 1939 and pertaining to: Determination of alcohol in the body fluids and tissues; metabolism of alcohol; effect of alcohol on bodily functions; nutritional diseases related to alcoholism; the alcoholic psychoses; treatment of the manifestations of alcoholism; and, statistical reports on alcohol consumption, alcohol and crime, accidents, mortality and morbidity. The article includes charts and tables and a 272-item bibliography.

Shipley, W. C. MEDICAL AND DOMESTIC USE OF WINE. *Med. Rec., 151:101–102.*

The paper deals with very general statements, alluding to the Bible, describing varieties of wine and their medical value. "Taken in moderation with food wine is refrigerant, stimulant, tonic and nutritive; it improves appetite, aids digestion, assimilation and elimination; it helps build up the blood, increasing its iron and hemoglobin, in simple anemias, and contributes to bodily well being." (p. 101)

1942

Thewlis, Malford W. THE CARE OF THE AGED (GERIATRICS). *St. Louis: The C. V. Mosby Company, Fourth edition. (First edition, 1919)*

A classic handbook on problems in geriatrics. In the section on therapeutic procedures, the author discusses alcohol, alcohol and food, general use of alcohol, its effect on the digestive apparatus, and cautions against abuse. "Alcohol is a narcotic and not a stimulant. It acts quickly and effectively in some neuralgic conditions and will often relieve gastric distress . . . Whisky, brandy, or wine usually will improve digestion if taken with meals." (pp. 143–144)

1943

Haggard, H. W.; L. A. Greenberg, and L. H. Cohen THE INFLUENCE OF THE CONGENERS OF DISTILLED SPIRITS UPON THE PHYSIOLOGICAL ACTION OF ALCOHOL. *Quart. J. Stud. Alc., 4:1–56.*

An article dealing with methods applicable to the study of the influence of congeners on beverage alcohol, specifically in distilled spirits.

Von Oettingen, W. F. THE ALIPHATIC ALCOHOLS: THEIR TOXICITY AND POTENTIAL DANGERS IN RELATION TO THEIR CHEMICAL CONSTITUTION AND THEIR FATE IN METABOLISM. *Public Health Bull. No. 281*

A monograph written by the principal industrial toxicologist, United States Public Health Service, which is in fact an extensive and critical review of the literature on the aliphatic alcohols. Appended is an excellent bibliography.

1944

Bertuzzi, Alberto IL VINO NELLA VOSTRA VITA. *Milan: A. Bertuzzi, Seventh edition.*

The author discusses types and storage of wine, and generalizes on the medicinal qualities of Italian wines. Appended is an index of Italian wines.

1948

Horwitz, O. CERTAIN PHARMACEUTICAL PROPERTIES OF ALCOHOL, NICOTINE AND CAFFEINE. *J. Aviation Med., 19:179–185.*

The author reports on the physiologic effects of alcohol on the human organism. With regard to the gastrointestinal tract, he states: "There seems to be no doubt . . . that large amounts of alcohol have serious effects both upon the function and upon the permanent condition of the mucosa of the stomach . . . However, if one has a healthy gastrointestinal tract, there is no reason to believe that small amounts of alcohol do anything but affect digestion favorably if taken with or before meals." (p. 180)

Mathé, C. P. WINE: ITS USE IN HEALTH AND DISEASE. *Med. Rec., 161:32–38.*

The author offers a rational approach to the use of wine as a source of food, to improve appetite, to facilitate digestion and as a sedative and tranquilizer.

1949

Richet, C. VIN ET ALCOOL EN DIETETIQUE. *Paris Méd., 39:581–583.*

Though condemning the high consumption of alcohol, the the author feels that many people, French in particular, develop a true physiological need for wine. He recommends dosages of wine and indicates where and how it should be used. "In hypochlorhydria, white wine may be used to stimulate secretion. In certain forms of anorexia we recommend white aperitif wines . . . some dyspeptics tolerate only white wines, others only red. In diarrhea a red wine rich in tannin is indicated." (p. 583)

1950

Reich, Philipp WEIN-KOMPENDIUM FÜR DEN ARZT. UEBERBLICK UND WEGWEISER. *Stuttgart: Wissenschaftliche Verlagsgesellschaft.*

A critical and detailed review in which the author discusses "all that is worth knowing about the chemical and physiological value of wine" and presents a rational approach to the therapeutic use of wine. The topics covered are: the chemistry of wine; physiologic and pharmacodynamic effect of wine; wine as an addictive drug; and the therapeutic uses of wine.

Stieglitz, E. J. NUTRITION PROBLEMS OF GERIATRIC MEDICINE. *J.A.M.A., 142:1070–1077.*

A clinical discussion of the problem of adequate diet in the geriatric patient. In the section on "Specific Nutritional Needs," the author states: "In my opinion the judicious use of whisky or other spiritus liquors is therefore indicated in the management of many aged patients. Alcohol in moderation supplies quick fuel, relaxes tensions and tends to increase the appetite. A glass of wine or a highball before dinner and another at bedtime is often most constructive in increasing vigor and endurance in the elderly." (p. 1077)

Tant, E. L'UTILITE DU VIN POUR LA SANTE DE L'HOMME. *Rev. Belge Vins et Spirit. (Abstract in: Bull. Int. Vin, 23:91–97.)*

The author describes the beneficial effects of wine in general terms, without specific substantiating evidence. "In small doses it [wine] warms the stomach and heart, and in drinking a glass of wine, one drinks a glass of joy, energy, health, and hope." (p. 96)

1952

Burbridge, T. N.; V. C. Sutherland, and C. R. Hine CONVERSION OF ETHANOL TO ACETALDEHYDE IN VITRO. *Fed. Proc., 11:328.*

The authors show that labeled acetaldehyde was recovered from labeled ethanol, indicating an important transformation occurring as a normal process in the metamorphosis of alcohol into both aromatic and saporific substances.

Sears, W. G. THE MEDICAL INDICATIONS FOR ALCOHOL. *Practitioner, 168:427–429.*

A brief review of the uses of alcohol, written by a clinician who considers such uses under three headings: therapeutic, dietetic, and convivial. "Used dietetically . . . the addition of a liquor suited to the palate of the individual may make all the difference between a distaste for meals and the ability to eat, assimilate and enjoy food." (p. 429)

1954
Flanzy, M.; J. Causeret, and D. Hugot ETAT PRESENT DE NOS
CONNAISSANCES SUR L'INTERET ALIMENTAIRE DU VIN. *Bull. Soc.
Sci. Hyg. Aliment., 42:84–112.*

An objective appraisal of the nutritional value of wine and
its physiologic effects, based on experimental data from the
literature and from the experiments of the authors. The topics
discussed are: Alcohol in wine (its utilization by the organism); is the effect of wine on the organism comparable to
that of an alcohol solution?; nutritional value of wine; constituents of wine, other than alcohol, which furnish energy; nitrogenous substances in wine; minerals; vitamins; the physiologic effects of wine; and, the influence of various oenologic
practices on the medicinal value of wine. In conclusion the
authors state that "in spite of the many publications, our
knowledge of the physiologic effect of wine remains incomplete. The best established facts concern the digestive system:
in general, wine stimulates salivary secretion and facilitates
gastric digestion of proteins; on the other hand it acts as an
excitant of the liver." (p. 110). Included is an extensive
bibliography.

Lucia, Salvatore P. WINE AS FOOD AND MEDICINE. *New York:
The Blakiston Company, Inc.*

A careful compilation of the literature on the physiologic
effects of wine on the human organism. The topics reviewed
are: the chemistry of wine; the physiologic effects of wine:
wine as food; the action of wine upon the digestive organs
and its use in diseases of the gastrointestinal tract; the action
of wine upon the respiratory system; the action of wine upon
the cardiovascular system; the action of wine upon the kidneys
and its use in renal disease; the action of wine upon the neuro-
muscular system; the use of wine in acute infectious diseases;
the use of wine in diabetes mellitus; wine as a vehicle for
medication; the use of wine in the treatment of the aged and
the convalescent; and a discussion on the elixir of the grape.
The contraindications to the therapeutic use of wine are listed
with each chapter.

1963
Lucia, Salvatore P. A HISTORY OF WINE AS THERAPY. WITH A
FOREWORD BY SANFORD V. LARKEY. *Philadelphia: J. B. Lippin-
cott Company.*

An historical saga of wine as an element of civilization. The book traces the use of wine in medicine by delving into the works of the great physicians: Hippocrates, Pliny, Galen, Maimonides, and so on, through Anstie, Yorke-Davies, Sir William Osler, into modern experimental medicine.

Also discussed are the medical uses of wine as outlined in such great books as the Bible; the Rig-Vedas; the Tantras; the Iliad and the Odyssey; Arnald's *Liber de vinis,* the *Regimen sanitatis salernitanum;* Trotula's *Diseases of Women;* Brunschwig's *The Vertuose Boke of Distyllacyon;* and such tracts as *The Juice of the Grape—or Wine Preferable to Water.*

The final chapter is "The Demonstration of the Physiologic Effects of Wine." In regard to the gastrointestinal system, the author states that, "After the pioneering work of Claude Bernard, scores of investigators in Europe and America conducted studies of the effects of alcohol on the digestive system. Most of them assumed, as the majority of reviewers still assume today, that the actions of various alcoholic beverages differ only according to the concentration of alcohol, thereby ignoring the sharp differences between the effects of plain solutions of alcohol and the effects of wine . . . Buchner, conducting experiments both *in vitro* and with human subjects, found that wines and malt beverages significantly retard the rate at which protein is digested, while alcohol in the same low concentrations does not. Similar results were reported a decade later by Sir William Roberts . . . [who] found, however, that while large quantities of wine, especially of sherry, retard proteolysis, small quantities of wine accelerate the process. He also demonstrated that dilute alcoholic solutions, including wines, stimulate the secretion of gastric juice and the muscular contractions of the stomach." (pp. 180–181)

Lucia, Salvatore Pablo, editor: ALCOHOL AND CIVILIZATION. *New York: McGraw-Hill Book Company, Inc.*

The published proceedings of a symposium designed, organized, and chaired by the editor, and held at the University of California School of Medicine, San Francisco, with an Introduction by John B. deC. M. Saunders, Dean of the School of Medicine.

Part 1 deals with *The Effects of Alcohol on the Body,* with reports on: Good-willed Judgment on Alcohol, by Chauncey D. Leake; The Metabolism of Alcohol, by Leonard Goldberg; Influence of Alcohol on the General Metabolism of the Body, by Olof A. Forsander; Alcohol in Relation to Dietary Patterns, by Claudia Balboni; The Clinical Value of Alcohol, by William Dock; and a panel discussion, Present Knowledge of the Physiology of Alcohol. Part 2 deals with *Alcohol and the Mind,* with reports on: Alcohol and Skilled Behavior, by George C. Drew; Alcohol and Emotional Behavior, by Leon A. Greenberg; Alcohol and Neurotic Behavior, by Jules H. Masserman; Alcohol and Behavioral Disorder—Alcoholism, by Franz Alexander; and a panel discussion, The Effects of Alcohol on Behavior and Emotion. Part 3 deals with *Social Implications of Alcohol,* with reports on: The Antiquity of Alcohol in Diet and Medicine, by Salvatore P. Lucia; Alcohol in Human Culture, by Bertron Roueché; The Cocktail Hour: Physiological, Psychological, and Social Aspects, by Giorgio Lolli; and a panel discussion, Alcohol in Contemporary Culture. Part 4 deals with *Alcohol in Our Society,* with reports on: To Drink or Not to Drink, by Robert Straus; Drinking Practices and Their Social Function, by Kettil Bruun; Alcohol and the Law, by John M. Murtagh; and a panel discussion, The Responsibility of the Individual and the Community. Parts 5 and 6 are panels, respectively on *Specific Viewpoints:* Clinical; Alcohol Intoxication; Psychological; and Sociological; and on *Interdisciplinary Viewpoints:* Psychology, Physiology, and Anthropology; Psychiatry, Nutrition, Physiology, and Literature; Medicine, Physiology, and Law; and Pharmacology, Medicine, and Psychology.

1965

Chafetz, Morris E. LIQUOR: THE SERVANT OF MAN. *Boston, Toronto: Little, Brown and Company.*

Written by a practicing psychiatrist and an authority on alcoholism, this book is a well-documented account of the historical use of alcohol and its beverages, presented with a minimum of prejudicial bias, together with modern interpretations of controversial issues.

Ritchie, J. M.: THE ALIPHATIC ALCOHOLS, *in* THE PHARMACOLOGICAL BASIS OF THERAPEUTICS. LOUIS S. GOODMAN AND ALFRED GILMAN, EDITORS. *New York: The Macmillan Company, Third edition, pp. 143–158 (First edition, 1941)*

In this text, the author gives a concise and authoritative scientific epitome of the physiologic effects of alcohol on the gastrointestinal tract. "The effects of various concentrations

and types of alcoholic beverages on the gastrointestinal motor
and secretory functions are influenced by a number of factors
. . . Gastric secretions, like salivary secretions, are usually
stimulated *psychically* by alcohol, especially if the individual
likes it. The gastric juice produced in this way [in the presence of alcohol in concentrations of about 10%] is rich in
acid and normal in pepsin content . . . It seems that temperate
ămounts [of alcoholic beverages] cannot be considered deleterious, and if one enjoys alcohol it may even affect digestion favorably if taken with meals." (p. 146)

Wendt, V. E., E. Wu; R. Balcon; G. Doty, and R. Bing HEMO-
DYNAMIC AND METABOLIC EFFECTS OF CHRONIC ALCOHOLISM IN
MAN. *Amer. J. Cardiol., 15:175–184.*

The authors showed that "frequent bouts of acute alcoholism might result in permanent alterations of metabolic pathways," disturbances of enzyme release and/or "alterations in
mitochondrial membrane permeability."

1966
Leake, Chauncey D., and Milton Silverman ALCOHOLIC BEVER-
AGES IN CLINICAL MEDICINE. *Chicago: Year Book Medical Pub-
lishers, Inc.*

A carefully documented epitome of the pharmacodynamic
effects of alcoholic beverages recommended for use in clinical
medicine. The work is systematically arranged and bears pertinent comments. A bibliography of 416 items is included.

Mackay, I. R. THE EFFECTS OF ALCOHOL ON THE GASTROINTES-
TINAL TRACT. *Med. J. Aust., 2:372–376.*

A prejudicial and non-critical random review article.

1968
Terhune, William B. THE SAFE WAY TO DRINK. HOW TO PRE-
VENT ALCOHOL PROBLEMS BEFORE THEY START. *William Mor-
row & Company, Inc.*

Written by a psychiatrist, this volume is controversial and
overtly prejudicial. The title is misleading in that it does not
insure the readers' avoidance of all the direful and equivocal
"terrors" the author levels at the use of alcoholic beverages.
The same logic could be applied to any substance used as food
or drink, and, therefore, the force of what the author wishes
to present is dissipated. The author's prohibitionist pretense at
a fair-minded exposition of the problem succeeds in accom-

plishing very little since the prejudices expressed against alcohol are given without tempered thought or scientific evidence.

1969

Lucia, Salvatore Pablo, editor: WINE AND HEALTH. *Menlo Park, Pacific Coast Publishers.*

Proceedings of the first International Symposium on Wine and Health, held at The University of Chicago Center for Continuing Education, November 9, 1968. An epitome of modern research concerning wine and its exposure to various chemical, clinical, and sociological disciplines.

Reports are included on: Wine and Tranquility, by Salvatore P. Lucia; Wine and Emotional Tension, by Leon A. Greenberg; The Uses of Wine in Diabetes Mellitus and Allied Disorders, by Giorgio Lolli; The Wondrous Constituents of Wine, by Pascal Ribéreau-Gayon; Biological Effects of Wine Pigments, by John J. Powers; The Place of Wine in the Care of Heart Disease, Cancer, and Stroke, by William Dock; and a panel discussion, The Use of Wine in Hospitals and Nursing Homes, by Robert Kastenbaum, Vincent C. Sarley, and Robert C. Stepto.

EFFECTS ON ABNORMAL FUNCTIONS

It is not our purpose to give a detailed description of the pathology of the digestive system. It should be stated however, that disorders of the gastrointestinal tract may involve predominantly one of its segments and be reflected in physiological dysfunction elsewhere. Occasionally symptoms are listed as pathological conditions, i.e., abdominal pain, diarrhea, constipation; these being the result of a disease involving a single organ, or of general malfunction of the digestive system with symptoms concentrated in one area. Observations and imputations by ancient as well as modern physicians indicate that wine exerts a positive psychologic and physiologic effect on the well-being and proper functioning of the digestive system.

Historically, wine—as most other ancient medicinal substances—has been used for its imputed effect as a palliative, alleviating or allaying agent. The results obtained, apparently specific but unexplained, have warranted the establishment of an empirical tradition with regard to the therapeutic use of local and regional wines for digestive disorders. It is realized that the psychological feature of illness yields, in a nonspecific way, to the euphorant, sedative and hypnotic properties of wine—or any other alcoholized dietary beverage. In general, the tendency has been to recommend a dry wine for anorexia, white wine for constipation, a wine high in tannin content for diarrhea, and iced sparkling wine for nausea. Though physicians usually prescribe wine orally, some recommend its administration by enema for the purpose of tanning the bowels, and also as an effective means of introducing nourishment where this becomes difficult because of continued nausea and vomiting. The proponents of regional wines exercise their prejudices by recommending the wines of their choice for special purposes. Thus Professor Rouget recommends the wines of the Jura "for persons who suffer from digestive troubles," while Professor Cayla recommends the wines of Bordeaux for gastritis, enteritis and entero-colitis.

Sir Humphrey Rolleston discussing situations where secretory and motor activity of the stomach is impaired, advises the use of beverage alcohol: "The good effect is not due solely to the alcohol, but also to the ethers contained in brandy and wines." Loeper and Lemaire found wine "more active than an equal quantity of alcohol diluted to a similar concentration," a finding later supported by studies on the bactericidal effect of wine.

In this section we shall list references dealing with the broad therapeutic use of wine in nonspecific diseases of the digestive system. Studies reporting the effect of wine in specific diseases will be discussed and incorporated in the appropriate subsections.

1855

Aran, A. F. DE L'EMPLOI DES LAVEMENTS DE VIN, EN PARTICULIER DANS LE TRAITEMENT DE LA CHLOROSE, DE LE DYSPEPSIE, DE LA PHTISIE PULMONAIRE, ETC., ET DANS LA CONVALESCENCE DES MALADIES GRAVES. *Bull. Thér., 48:10–14.*

Three case histories are presented in which wine was administered rectally with very good results. This route was chosen because of the inability of the patient to retain food, or because of hypersensitivity of upper segments of the gastrointestinal tract. The subjects suffered from long-standing severe diarrhea, acute gastroenteritis, and pulmonary tuberculosis.

1859

Ollier, L. F. A. ESSAI D'OENOLOGIE MEDICALE. *Strasbourg: Thesis #466.*

The author discusses the use of wine both externally as well as internally. Concerning the external therapeutic effects of wine, he cites its use in lotions, fumigations, in the treatment of wounds, ulcers, and reports the recommendation of Stoltz regarding antisepsis of female genitals after delivery as well as of the newborn infant. Referable to the gastrointestinal tract, the author recommends enemas of lightly astringent wine—old Bordeaux being preferable—in chronic and atonic diarrhea.

1880

Rouget, P. M. J. V. ESSAI MEDICAL SUR LES VINS DU JURA. *Paris: Thesis #17.*

The author quotes Doctor Nonat who suggests a small glass of the regional wine after each meal "for persons who suffer from digestive troubles." (p. 85)

1907

Cayla, F. REGIMES PATHOLOGIQUES ET REGIME PARFAIT. *Paris: Vigot frères.*

In diseases of the digestive system, such as gastritis, enteritis, entero-colitis, the author recommends, "with the evening meal Bordeaux wine, red in winter and white in summer, generously diluted with water." (p. 44)

1913

Fiessinger, Charles VINGT REGIMES ALIMENTAIRES EN CLIENTELE. *Paris: A. Maloine.*

A collection of dietary regimens for various diseases, extolling the use of wine in its various dosages.

Hutchison, R. DISCUSSION ON THE VALUE OF ALCOHOL AS A THERAPEUTIC AGENT. *Roy. Soc. Med. Proc. (Sect. Ther. & Pharmacol.), 13:46–47.*

The author expresses his opinion that alcohol "is a digestive stimulant and is often useful in cases of impaired appetite, gastric atony and in convalescence. The form in which it is administered has, however, a great influence on its digestive value." (p. 46)

1921

Mallory, W. J. EFFECT OF ALCOHOL ON THE GASTROINTESTINAL TRACT. *Med. Rec., 100:275–277.*

A lecture read before the American Therapeutic Association. The therapeutic uses of beverage alcohol in diseases of the gastrointestinal tract are discussed.

Stockton, C. G. EFFECT OF ALCOHOL IN THERAPY OF INTERNAL DISEASES. *Med. Rec., 100:277–279.*

The author reviews the circumstances under which alcohol can be used with beneficial results. "In old age . . . there can be no doubt of the very great importance of alcohol. Used judiciously and with the same care which is exercised in the prescription of other drugs, alcohol often enables an aged person to live on, not only with greater functional power, but with comparative satisfaction . . ." (p. 278)

1924

Rolleston, Sir H. ALCOHOL IN MEDICINE. *Practitioner, 113:209–215.*

One of a series of articles devoted to alcohol in which the author, physician to the King of England, gives "a brief consideration of the much debated value of alcohol in medical treatment." With regard to the gastrointestinal tract, he states: "In cases of convalescence from acute disease, when the secretory and motor activities of the stomach are impaired, . . . the addition of alcohol . . . to the meals may make all the difference between distaste for meals and painful digestion on the one hand, and ability both to eat and assimilate food on the other hand. The good effect is not due solely to the alcohol, but also to the contained ethers in brandy and wines, . . . In flatulence a small dose of a concentrated alcoholic drink, such as old brandy or a liqueur, may act like a charm in relieving the 'windy spasm.' " (pp. 213–214)

1930

Loeper, Maurice, and André Lemaire THERAPEUTIQUE MEDICALE. I. MALADIES DU TUBE DIGESTIF. *Paris: Masson et Cie.*

The authors discuss diseases of the digestive tract and give directions for the use of wine in certain cases. "When painful indigestion is present, pepsin should be administered in *vin ordinaire,* providing that it does not exceed 2 per cent by volume . . . Wine is more active than an equal quantity of alcohol diluted to the same concentration; that is, natural wine since adulterated wines contain inhibitory substances which injure the mucosa." (pp. 89, 96)

1935

Soresi, A. L. WINE ENEMA AND PROCTOCLYSIS. *Med. Rec., 141:435.*

A discussion on the advantages of wine enemas, pre- and post-operatively. The author recommends a port-type wine (ca. 20% alcohol) pre-operatively, and Angelica, or similar type wine, post-operatively. He considers wine by proctoclysis "favorable for the induction of anesthesia," and states that it lessens considerably the amount of anesthetic required. Furthermore, he found that preliminary medication with opiates was unnecessary.

1937

Serianni, E. LE VIN ET LE JUS DE RAISIN DANS LE DIETETIQUE ET DANS LE TRAITEMENT DES AFFECTIONS GASTRO-INTESTINALES. *IVe Congrès Nat'l. Méd. Amis des Vins de France, Alger, pp. 58–68.*

Weissenbach, R. J., and G. Faroy LE VIN ET LE JUS DE RAISIN DANS LA DIETETIQUE ET LE TRAITEMENT DES AFFECTIONS GAS-TRO-INTESTINALES. *IVe Congrès Nat'l Méd. Amis des Vins de France, Alger, pp. 86–158.*

A monograph in which the various constituents of wine are discussed and its physiologic effects elaborated. The main theme is the use of wine in diseases of the digestive tract, including specific contraindications. The conclusions of the authors and their specific recommendations will be found in the appropriate subsections.

1939

Sorel, R. LES QUALITES THERAPEUTIQUES DU VIN. *Conf. d'Oenologie Fac. Méd. Toulouse, pp. 60–67.*

The author discusses the following specific constituents of wine: ethyl alcohol, sugars, pectins and resins, salts and vitamins. Included is a description of some of the medicinal wines and a suggested list of specific wines in specific diseases. "In diseases of the gastrointestinal tract . . . red wines rich in tannin in cases of diarrhea, . . . soft white wines in constipation, . . . white wines or 'Rancio' wines in hypochlorhydric dyspepsias, . . . iced champagnes or sparkling wines in severe vomiting." He further enumerates gastrointestinal diseases in which wine should be prohibited.

1942

McGee, L. C., and J. D. Creger GASTROINTESTINAL DISEASE AMONG INDUSTRIAL WORKERS. *J.A.M.A., 120:1367–1369.*

1963

Lucia, Salvatore P. WINE AS FOOD AND MEDICINE. *New York: The Blakiston Company, Inc.*

"Wine is widely used in the treatment of diseases of the digestive system. It is found to be particularly beneficial in anorexia, hypochlorhydria without gastritis and hyposthenic dyspepsia. Minor hepatic insufficiency responds not unfavorably to unadulterated dry white table wine. The tannin content and the mildly antiseptic properties of wine make it valuable in the treatment of intestinal colic, mucous colitis, spastic constipation, diarrhea and many infectious diseases of the gastrointestinal tract. By virtue of the anesthetic effect of carbon dioxide, champagne or effervescent wines give excellent results in prolonged nausea and in vomiting caused by gastric irritation." (p. 56)

CONTRAINDICATIONS

There is no evidence that wine in reasonable quantities will adversely affect the healthy gastrointestinal tract. The consensus seems to be that "if one has a healthy gastrointestinal tract, there is no reason to believe that small amounts of alcohol do anything but affect digestion favorably if taken with or before meals." (see Horwitz, 1948) An important study which may indicate a noxious effect of wine on the functional state of the stomach was carried out in 1833 by William Beaumont who felt that the acidity in wine in combination with its alcohol content is injurious to the gastric mucosa.

1833
Beaumont, William EXPERIMENTS AND OBSERVATIONS ON THE GASTRIC JUICE AND THE PHYSIOLOGY OF DIGESTION. *Plattsburgh: F. P. Allen.*

Written by a surgeon in the United States Army and a "pioneer American physiologist," the work is divided into two main sections. In the first section is discussed: aliments, hunger and thirst, satisfaction and satiety, mastication, insalivation and deglutition, gastric digestion, chylification and uses of the bile and pancreatic juice. The second part of the book comprises an account of four series of experiments and observations on one male subject who, as a result of a gunshot wound, developed partial protrusion of the stomach (gastric fistula). At the end of the book the author states his conclusions. "The injury which a constant use of wine is known to produce on some stomachs, has been sometimes attributed to the small quantity of tartaric acid which it [wine] contains. But . . . it is the acidity . . . contained in the wine, aided, perhaps, by the alcohol which is in a state of combination with it [which is responsible for the injury to the stomach mucosa.]" (p. 50)

1880
Samson, G. W. THE DIVINE LAW AS TO WINES; ESTABLISHED BY THE TESTIMONY OF SAGES, PHYSICIANS, AND LEGISLATORS AGAINST THE USE OF FERMENTED AND INTOXICATING WINES; CONFIRMED BY THEIR PROVISION OF UNFERMENTED WINES TO BE USED FOR MEDICINAL AND SACRAMENTAL PURPOSES. *New York: The National Temperance Society and Publication House.*

An analysis of the Bible which purports to demonstrate that the reference to wine concerns the unfermented juice of the grape, and where an intoxicating drink is discussed it is usually warned against and found unfit for use by the "princes of the land." It is an earnest, but one-sided, defense of prohibition on religious grounds. "All medical and chemical authorities agree that pure alcohol is a most active poison; excoriating and deadening when applied externally to the skin; and yet more active and deadly when received inwardly upon the delicate membranes of the mouth, throat, and stomach." (p. 37)

1965
Goodman, Louis S., and Alfred Gilman, editors THE PHARMACOLOGICAL BASIS OF THERAPEUTICS. *New York: The Macmillan Company, Third edition.*

"[Alcohol is contraindicated in] ulceration of the gastrointestinal tract and hyperacidity associated with digestive complaints." (p. 146)

2

The Effects of Wine and its Constituents on the Functions and Disorders of the Upper Gastrointestinal Tract

EFFECTS ON NORMAL FUNCTIONS

The initial steps in the digestive process take place in the mouth where the food is broken down by the chewing action of the teeth and attacked by the enzymatic action of the saliva. Although the mouth and salivary glands are considered accessory organs of the gastrointestinal tract, and the teeth are actually part of the skeleton, they are nonetheless important parts of the digestive system.

The pharynx is the section of the digestive system which shares some of its functions with the respiratory system—it is the common vestibule for commestibles and air. The esophagus connects the mouth and pharynx with the alimentary organs of the abdominal cavity. No digestive activity occurs in the esophagus, nor does any absorption take place there under normal circumstances. Wine, like other liquids, apparently only moistens the mucous membranes of these organs.

The grinding surface of the teeth—their enamel crowns—are almost entirely calcific in composition. That wine contributes anything to dental health is unknown. As there is very little direct interchange between the calcium of the body and that of the dental crowns, the contents of calcium in wine would bear no relevance to the structure of the teeth, excepting under circumstances of powerfully ionizable acids. The tannin content of wine, however, may have a salubrious and therapeutic effect in conditions where constriction of gingival tissues is desirable.

Saliva consists mainly of water harboring dilute solutions of proteinaceous materials including enzymes, and a small amount of inorganic salts (less than 1%). It is secreted by the buccal glands—parotid, sublingual, and submaxillary. The salivary enzyme ptyalin is responsible for converting starch into a simple sugar, while salivary bicarbonate provides the required degree of alkalinity.

Considerable attention has been devoted to the effect of wine on the salivary glands and salivary secretion. Roberts, Billings, and Starling found that wine inhibits salivary secretion, and they ascribe this inhibition to the acidity of wine. Chittenden, Horsley, and Bravo, on the other hand, are of the opinion that wine not only increases the volume of salivary secretion but also its digestive propensities. There have been some pertinent studies carried out on the relationship between olfactory acuity, appetite, and hunger. Goetzl found that wine increases olfactory acuity, and Haggard and Jellinek noted that when alcohol in moderation reaches the stomach, it is capable of stimulating hunger and that this effect can be achieved also by intravenous injections of alcohol.

In relation to the olfactory sense, the role of aroma and bouquet of wine must be given special consideration. Bouquet is the combination of, and interplay between, aroma and flavor of a wine. This subtle blending epitomizes the amalgamation and the mellowing of the saporific substances and their odors.

The sense of smell is directly or indirectly responsible for many of our reactions of appreciation. New foods are often accepted or rejected solely on the basis of odor. The area responsible for the perception of smell is the nasopharynx. One might say that the nose is the receptor and the pharynx the vestibule in which wine paves the way for the organs of taste to appreciate its bouquet, and the professional wine-taster is thus left to dream about an organized marriage of these two senses.

Taste is a matter of four attributes—sweet, sour, salt and bitter. The flavor of what we taste is altered by the odoroforic perception of aroma within the nose. By combining the sense of taste with that of smell we broaden our awareness and are thus enabled to recognize an infinite variety of aromas.

Having discussed the importance of taste and smell in relation to wine, we must now introduce the role of the psyche. It is generally accepted that sight and smell, memory and anticipation of a food can stimulate appetite and initiate salivary secretion. It is also accepted that loss of appetite may be due to the conflicting psychologic features of tension or depression. The effect of wine on appetite is mediated through its pharmacodynamic activity which apparently stimulates the taste apparatus physiologically, and ultimately enhances appetite by removing tensions through its qualities as a tranquilizer. There is experimental evidence that wine excites the papillae of the tongue, and some investigators believe that it has a direct action upon the nerve endings in the buccal cavity and its organelles. Pavlov, Starling, Himwich, and many other investigators have found that wine effectively initiates appetite either by stimulating the gustatory papillae or by virtue of its tranquilizing action. Wine, they state, is most valuable in the treatment of certain types of anorexia.

Since the stomach and its gastric secretions may well play a prominent role in the sensation known as appetite, papers and books referring to this effect of wine on appetite will be included in this account.

1568
Turner, William A BOOK OF WINES . . . *New York: Scholars' Facsimiles and Reprints, 1941.*

"Generally every wine not mixed . . . maketh a man have an appetite." (p. 47)

1824
Kitchiner, William: THE ART OF INVIGORATING AND PROLONGING LIFE . . . *London: Hurst, Robinson, and Co., Fifth edition.*

"Undiluted [port and sherry] are too strong to be drunk during Dinner,—they act so powerfully on the feelings of the Stomach, that they dull the desire for solid Food." (p. 161)

1877
Anstie, Francis E. ON THE USES OF WINES IN HEALTH AND DISEASE. *London: Macmillan and Co.*

". . . the useful functions of such quantities of free acids as are found in natural wines are limited to their tonic stimulant action upon stomach-digestion. And that this must be a powerful action no one will doubt who has systematically observed the effects of acid (but otherwise sound) wines in restoring appetite (p. 23) . . . A moderate amount of *astringency* perhaps may increase somewhat the good effects of such wines upon the appetite; . . . (p. 64)

1886
Roberts, Sir William LECTURES ON DIETETICS AND DYSPEPSIA. *London: Smith, Elder & Co., Second edition.*

In the second lecture, Sir William, describing experiments with wine on salivary digestion states: "Both the stronger and the lighter wines showed a powerful inhibitory effect on salivary digestion . . . The inhibitory effect of wines is entirely due to the very considerable degree of acidity which they all possess." (p. 25)

Yeo, J. B. FOOD ACCESSORIES; THEIR INFLUENCE ON DIGESTION. *Nineteenth Century, 19:271–279.*

The author is of the opinion that diluted alcohol, in moderate doses, increases the flow of saliva and promotes digestion. In the form of brandy or whiskey, alcohol interferes with digestion. A solution of alcohol of 10% or less did not appreciably retard digestion and only a slight retardation occurred with a solution of 20%. But with higher concentration, "the digestive ferment was almost paralyzed." (p. 273)

1898
Chittenden, R. H.; L. B. Mendel, and H. C. Jackson A FURTHER STUDY OF THE INFLUENCE OF ALCOHOL AND ALCOHOLIC DRINKS UPON DIGESTION, WITH SPECIAL REFERENCE TO SECRETION. *Amer. J. Physiol., 1:164–209.*

"Upon the secretion of saliva, the presence of strong alcohol or an alcoholic beverage in the mouth has a direct stimulating effect leading to a sudden increase in the flow of saliva . . . This . . . however, is of brief duration. The stimulating effect is manifested not only by an increase in the volume of secretion, but also by an increase in both organic and inorganic constituents." (p. 207)

1903
Billings, John S. PHYSIOLOGICAL ASPECTS OF THE LIQUOR PROBLEM. *New York: Houghton, Mifflin and Company, 2 vols.*

"When alcohol and alcoholic beverages are taken into the mouth, there is a direct stimulating effect upon the secretion of mixed saliva, increasing at once and in a very marked degree the flow of secretion . . . The stimulating effect of alcohol is manifested . . . also by an increase in the proportion of both organic and inorganic constituents [of the salivary secretion] . . . With active saliva not greatly diluted the presence of even five per cent of absolute alcohol . . . may lead to a slight increase in digestive power . . . Wines, as a class, show a very powerful inhibitory influence upon salivary digestion, an influence which is due almost entirely to their acid properties." (Vol. 1, pp. 152, 154)

1909
Horsley, Sir Victor, and Mary D. Sturge ALCOHOL AND THE HUMAN BODY . . . *London: Macmillan and Co., Limited.*

"Like any other irritant, alcohol when in the mouth stimulates the nerves, and, by reflex action, causes an extra secretion of saliva. Now this extra flow of saliva due to the action of alcohol is not needful to the economy, because food when taken into the mouth and kept there a reasonable time calls forth a supply of saliva adequate to the purposes of preliminary digestion . . . As the 'bouquet' of a good vintage provides a pleasant momentary stimulus to the palate, it may reflexly cause secretory activity . . . but we believe that pleasure of such a kind will be relinquished by many in proportion as knowledge spreads regarding the close association between alcohol and disease." (pp. 183, 206)

1910
Pavlov, I. P. THE WORK OF THE DIGESTIVE GLANDS, LECTURES BY PROFESSOR I. P. PAVLOV. TRANSLATED INTO ENGLISH BY W. H. THOMPSON. *London: C. Griffin & Company, Limited. Second English edition. (First English edition, 1902)*

A collection of lectures delivered at St. Petersburg and first published in Russian in 1897. In the fourth lecture of this volume, the author discusses the significance of "psychic or appetite juice in the secretory work of the stomach" wherein he stresses the importance of sensory stimulation of appetite. This, he feels, may be achieved either by physiological or psychological means. Among the psychological stimuli he classified the ritual of the dinner hour: the changing into non-working clothes, soft lights, tabu on discussing business, and the serving of a beverage alcohol. Discussing the effect of some of these on appetite, he states: "After an illness . . . on the second or third day [I endeavoured] to create an appetite by swallowing a mouthful of wine. I felt it quite distinctly pass into . . . my stomach, and literally at that moment perceived the onset of a keen appetite." (p. 109)

1921

Mallory, W. J. EFFECT OF ALCOHOL ON THE GASTROINTESTINAL TRACT. *Med. Rec., 100:275–277.*

"Alcoholic beverages containing aromatic substances . . . act through the end organs of taste to increase appetite . . . In any case, where it is desired to awaken or stimulate the appetite, one of the wines or malted [fermented] drinks would be an aid." (p. 277)

1923

Starling, Ernest H. THE ACTION OF ALCOHOL ON MAN . . . *London: Longmans, Green and Co.*

In the section on digestion, the author states: "When dilute alcohol or alcoholic beverages are taken into the mouth they cause an increased flow of saliva . . . Not only is the amount of saliva increased, but there is an increase also in its solid contents and its starch digesting powers . . . If instead of using alcohol we use beverages such as spirits or wines, a marked retarding influence may be observed, but this is due solely to their acid properties and may be abolished by neutralizing the fluids . . ." (pp. 109–110).

1924

Starling, E. H. THE PHYSIOLOGICAL ACTION OF ALCOHOL. *Practitioner, 113:226–235.*

An article reviewing the metabolism of alcohol, the food value of alcohol, its action on the central nervous system, on digestion, on respiration, and on heat regulation. With regard to digestion, the author states: "The value of wine with a meal is chiefly as an appetizer, i.e., is due to its effects on the central nervous system. Anything which adds to the enjoyment or to the anticipated enjoyment of a meal, or to the removal of disturbing states of mind . . . will increase the appetite and be favorable to the normal process of digestion. [However,] strong alcohol, i.e., over 12 to 15 per cent, acts as an irritant to the mucous membranes . . ." (p. 234)

1932

Cambiaire, Célestin Pierre THE BLACK HORSE OF THE APOCALYPSE. (WINE, ALCOHOL, AND CIVILIZATION.) *Paris: Librairie*

Universitaire J. Gamber.

An extensive, well-documented but not always discerning, refutation of prohibition, dealing mainly with the social and economic implications of this legislation. One section is devoted to the role of alcoholic beverages in health and disease. On the use of wines as appetizers, the author states: "Even supposing that their influence would be merely imaginary their use would be justified since imagination has much to do with the nerves that control digestion." (p. 21)

Schram, C. F. N. LIQUOR FROM THE MEDICAL POINT OF VIEW. *Industr. Med., 1:114–117.*

An article reviewing the major physiologic effects of alcohol, but stressing the consequences of abuse and chronic use of alcohol. The author comments on appetite: "Taken by mouth, in moderation and properly diluted, alcoholic drinks tend to improve the appetite and give a feeling of warmth and comfort in the stomach, and to promote the digestive functions." (p. 114)

Webb, W. W.; R. B. Mullenix, and C. A. Dragstedt ABSORPTION OF DRUGS FROM THE ESOPHAGUS. *Proc. Soc. Exp. Biol. Med., 29:895–897.*

These authors are of the opinion that absorption from the esophagus can take place when: 1) the latter has been irritated or damaged by the passage of concentrated solutions of alcohol, or 2) when there has been impairment of the emptying mechanism.

1933

Winsor, A. L., and E. I. Strongin THE EFFECT OF ALCOHOL ON THE RATE OF PAROTID SECRETION. *J. Exp. Psychol., 16:589–597.*

A method for measuring parotid secretion is described. This study indicates that alcohol may be classed as a stimulant of parotid secretion only when it is in actual contact with the end organs within the wall of the digestive tract. Once the alcohol passes into the blood stream, its action is definitely inhibitory.

1934

Bravo, J. EFFETS DU VIN DANS LES PROCESSUS DIGESTIFS. *IIe Congrès Nat'l. Méd. Amis des Vins de France, Béziers, pp. 297–301.*

The author reviews the physiological effects of wine on digestion. He states that wine augments the salivary secretion reflexly and psychically by its direct action on glandular tissue. Wine, he states, "favors the digestion of carbohydrates . . ." (p. 299)

Dontas, S. L'ACTION PHYSIOLOGIQUE DU VIN SUR L'ORGANISME. *Bull. Int. Vin, 7:80–82.*

A review of data presented by various authors on the physiologic action of alcohol, incorporating some of the author's medical experiences with alcohol, notably wine. Referable to appetite, he says: "By its taste and its direct action on the mucous membranes of the buccal cavity, good wine provokes an abundant reflex secretion of saliva." (p. 80)

1936

Cruess, W. V. WINE IN THE DIET. *Fruit Prod. J., 15:260.*

The author is of the opinion that one of the most easily demonstrable effects of wine is that of stimulating appetite.

1937

Weissenbach, R. J., and G. Faroy LE VIN ET LE JUS DE RAISIN DANS LA DIETETIQUE ET LE TRAITEMENT DES AFFECTIONS GASTRO-INTESTINALES. *IVe Congrès Natl. Méd. Amis des Vins de France, Alger, pp. 86–158.*

Wine "releases salivary secretions which certain authors consider as the beginning of the sensation known as appetite . . . Primarily, wine excites the gustatory papillae . . . This is followed by an abundant flow of salivary secretion rich in ptyalin." (pp. 97–98)

1938

Scott, C. C.; W. W. Scott, and A. B. Luckhardt THE EFFECT OF ALCOHOL ON THE HUNGER SENSE. *Amer. J. Physiol., 123:248–255.*

Report of experiments on human subjects, describing a method of recording the intensity of hunger contractions after the ingestion of 200 cc. of a 20% solution of alcohol and the same amount of water (control). Alcohol caused some delay in onset of hunger, but had no effect on the amplitude of the contractions. Hunger sensations with alcohol were 105% more intense, on the average, than with water. The sensation produced was associated with an increased desire for food, but was less intense than hunger, and continuous; consequently it was considered to be "appetite."

1939

Emerson, Haven ALCOHOL AND MAN. THE EFFECTS OF ALCOHOL ON MAN IN HEALTH AND DISEASE. *New York: The Macmillan Company. (First edition, 1932)*

A collection of articles written by physiologists, pharmacologists, physicians, and other students of the life sciences, who base their statements on scientific data and on personal observations.

Brooks, Harlow: "Alcohol so used as a food may stimulate the appetite, unless given as it should only very rarely be, in a concentrated form; it increases the flow of the digestive juices from the mouth to the colon, but without increasing the digestive capacities of these products." (p. 163)

Himwich, Harold E.: "It is a general belief that alcoholic beverages improve the appetite and digestion . . . It may be that the beneficial effect on the appetite is an indirect result of the narcotic action of alcohol on the higher functions of the brain. By procuring release from worries and inhibitions, it may create the better spirits which are conducive to the efficient digestion of food." (p. 20)

Hyman, Harold Thomas: "Many factors qualify the response of the secreting surface of the gastro-intestinal tract to an average dose of alcohol which has been taken as a beverage . . . The irritation of the alcohol itself will definitely stimulate salivary and gastric secretion. In the latter instance, both the mucus and acid of the stomach will be increased." (p. 69)

Wallace, George B.: ". . . in concentrations under 10%, alcohol brings about a marked increase in gastric secretion. The secretion appears promptly and continues for some time, two hours or more. It comes when alcohol is given alone or when it is given with food. The increased secretion is not of normal composition, however, for while it contains hydrochloric acid in the usual proportion, the ferment pepsin is either actually or relatively diminished." (p. 35)

1940

Beazell, J. M., and A. C. Ivy THE INFLUENCE OF ALCOHOL ON THE DIGESTIVE TRACT. *Quart. J. Stud. Alc., 1:45–73.*

"Alcohol by exciting sensory nerve endings in the mouth reflexly stimulates a flow of saliva which is followed by a poststimulatory depression of secretion . . . The increase in appetite ascribed to alcoholic beverages is apparently due to the stimulation of the end organs of taste and general sensibility, . . . or to a central effect, such as promotion of the feeling of well-being, both of which affect the appetite mechanism." (pp. 68–69)

1942

Haggard, Howard W., and E. M. Jellinek ALCOHOL EXPLORED. *Garden City, New York: Doubleday, Doran & Company, Inc.*

A book in which some of the physiological effects of alcohol are discussed, but which concerns itself mainly with the excessive or abnormal use of alcohol, its social implications, and means of prevention of abuses. On appetite, the authors state: "It has long been observed that moderate amounts of alcoholic beverages taken before meals increase the desire for food . . . When alcohol, diluted with water to 20.0 per cent, was drunk by a fasting man the hunger contractions that were occurring were stopped for a short time as they would be by any food or fluid; during this time, however, a vague and continuous sensation was felt over the region of the stomach and was associated with a desire for food. When the hunger contractions started again, their actual force was no greater than before the alcohol was taken, but they were felt as stronger. Thus it would appear that moderate amounts of alcohol actually increase the sensations that are experienced as a desire for food." (p. 100)

1945

Haggard, H. W. THE PHYSIOLOGICAL EFFECTS OF LARGE AND SMALL AMOUNTS OF ALCOHOL, IN: ALCOHOL, SCIENCE AND SOCIETY. *New Haven: Quarterly Journal of Studies on Alcohol, pp. 59–72.*

A lecture delivered at the Yale Summer School of Alcohol Studies, describing briefly the physiological effects and the possible medicinal use of alcoholic beverages. On appetite, the author states: "Alcohol in moderate amounts leads to an increase in the flow of gastric juice and to contraction of the stomach. The sensation of hunger may develop. These changes occur when alcohol is administered intravenously as well as by mouth and are therefore not due solely to a local action on the stomach." (pp. 66–67)

1949

McCarthy, Raymond G., and Edgar M. Douglass ALCOHOL AND SOCIAL RESPONSIBILITY. A NEW EDUCATIONAL APPROACH. *New York: Thomas Y. Crowell Company and Yale Plan Clinic.*

A sociologic study which "has been prepared in response

to thousands of requests addressed to the Yale Plan on Alcoholism for an objective treatment of the problems of alcohol based on scientific facts." It discusses the problems and pertinent scientific data in non-technical terminology. In the appendix, information is given on private organizations concerned with education on alcohol and alcoholism. In the section on the physiologic effects of alcohol, the authors state: "Alcoholic beverages in the form of wines or beer consumed with certain foods, and cordials taken after dinner, have an appeal for many people. There may be some slight increase in the flow of gastric juice resulting from the ingestion of small amounts of beverages with a low alcoholic content, and this may intensify appetite." (p. 108)

1950

Goetzl, F. R. HUMAN APPETITE. *Permanente Found. Med. Bull., 8:72–86.*

A lecture presented at the University of California (Davis) in which the author gives definitions for "appetite" and "hunger," and then reviews the work his research group has done with regard to appetite. He discusses the effect of milk, bitter tonics, sugar, alcohol and wine on appetite.

Irvin, D. L.; A. J. Ahokas, and F. R. Goetzl THE INFLUENCE OF ETHYL ALCOHOL IN LOW CONCENTRATIONS UPON OLFACTORY ACUITY AND THE SENSATION COMPLEX OF APPETITE AND SATIETY. *Permanente Found. Med. Bull., 8:97–106.*

Experiments are described in which it is shown that the lowest concentration at which ethyl alcohol has to be ingested by normal individuals, in order to produce simultaneously a decrease in olfactory acuity and a conversion of the sensation of appetite into one of satiety, varies from 3.0 to 5.0 per cent alcohol.

Margulies, N. R.; D. L. Irvin, and F. R. Goetzl THE EFFECT OF ALCOHOL UPON OLFACTORY ACUITY AND THE SENSATION COMPLEX OF APPETITE AND SATIETY. *Permanente Found. Med. Bull., 8:1–8.*

Experiments on human subjects are described indicating that alcohol is capable of bringing about simultaneously a decrease in olfactory acuity and a conversion of the sensation of appetite into one of satiety. The relationship between olfactory acuity and the sensation complex of appetite and satiety is discussed.

1951

Irvin, D. L., and F. R. Goetzl THE INFLUENCE OF TANNIC ACID UPON OLFACTORY ACUITY AND THE SENSATION COMPLEX OF APPETITE AND SATIETY. *Permanente Found. Med. Bull., 9:119–124.*

A further report on the experimental work on appetite and satiety. Experiments are described indicating that tannic acid ingested during meals is capable of simultaneously preventing postcibal decrease in olfactory acuity and of interfering in the creation of the sensation of satiety. The suggestion is made that this effect of tannic acid may be related to the appetite-stimulating effect commonly ascribed to bitter tonics.

Janowitz, H. D., and M. I. Grossman EFFECT OF PREFEEDING ALCOHOL AND BITTERS ON FOOD INTAKE OF DOGS. *Amer. J. Physiol., 164:182–186.*

A report on experiments carried out on six dogs which were given 15 to 60 cc. of 50% alcohol 20 minutes before their regular feeding time over a period of several weeks. No change in their food intake was noted.

1953

Irvin, D. L.; A. Durra, and F. R. Goetzl INFLUENCE OF TANNIC, TARTARIC AND ACETIC ACID UPON OLFACTORY ACUITY AND SENSATIONS ASSOCIATED WITH FOOD INTAKE. *Amer. J. Dig. Dis., 20:17–21.*

One of a series of experimental studies which show that tannic, tartaric and acetic acid ingested during meals can simultaneously prevent postcibal decrease in olfactory acuity and interfere with satiety. The authors are of the opinion that this may be related to the appetite-stimulating effect of dry wines and bitter tonics.

1965

Goodman, Louis S., and Alfred Gilman, editors THE PHARMACOLOGICAL BASIS OF THERAPEUTICS. *New York: The Macmillan Company, Third edition.*

"Alcoholic beverages, if enjoyed by the patient, may be given before meals as a *stomachic* to improve appetite and digestion, especially in convalescent and debilitated or elderly patients." (p. 152)

EFFECTS ON ABNORMAL FUNCTIONS

Within the domain of disorders of the gastrointestinal tract, there are relatively few which could be considered primarily oral; among these are stomatitis and aphthous disorders. The effect of wine in these conditions has rarely been recorded, but the German physician Loebenstein-Loebel (1817) reported that "in the third stage of aphthae, we have obtained good results by touching them with burgundy wine two or three times daily."

The pharynx and esophagus are protected from many diseases by their tough membranous tissue. Mechanical disabilities, such as dysphagia, may occur as a result of a variety of esophageal obstructions and, despite the toughness of the esophageal wall, ulcers may occur here. While there is no evidence that wine has any curative effects in such conditions, it is suggested that when the mechanical passage of solid foods is impaired, maintenance of nutrition may be facilitated by the judicious use of wine. Labbé (1917) recommends "a little wine or a few drops of cognac in milk . . . in affections of the esophagus."

Although anorexia is a symptom complex of many systemic diseases, it is nonetheless included here because marked loss of appetite could result in grave deficiencies which might impair the normal functions of the gastrointestinal tract. Many physicians, realizing the stimulating effect of wine on salivary secretion and aware of its tranquilizing effect, have recommended wine for anorexia. Dr. Reich (1950) states that "there is no drug which can replace wine in the constant fight against loss of appetite."

1817
Loebenstein-Loebel, Ed. TRAITE SUR L'USAGE ET LES EFFETS DES VINS. *Strasbourg: F. G. Levrault.*

". . . in the third state of aphthae, we have obtained good results by touching them [the lesions] with burgundy wine two or three times daily." (p. 52)

1866
Fonssagrives, J. B. THERAPEUTIQUE DE LA PHTISIE PULMONAIRE BASEE SUR LES INDICATIONS, OU L'ART DE PROLONGER LA VIE DES PHTISIQUES PAR LES RESSOURCES COMBINEES DE L'HYGIENE ET DE LA MATIERE MEDICALE. *Paris: J. B. Baillière et fils.*

A very extensive and well-documented handbook on the care of pulmonary tuberculosis. Many aspects of treatment and prevention of the disease are discussed; one section is devoted to dietary considerations. In anorexia associated with tuberculosis, "wine of chinchona [extract of chinchona dissolved in red wine] is commonly used as an aperitif; but, in order to avoid digestive disturbances and to obtain the most beneficial effect, it should be taken with the meal; never on an empty stomach." (p. 375)

1880

THE LANCET COMMISSION ON THE MEDICAL USE OF WINES. *Lancet, 1:1001–1003.*

Report of a commission established to study the therapeutic value of wine shortly after Gladstone's campaign to raise import duties on the cheaper and lighter French wines. In this report only the white wines of Bordeaux are discussed. When reporting on the effect of wine on appetite, the Commission states: ". . . thin [white] wines, with less body and flavour, and a slightly acidulous taste . . . excite the appetite, [and] may be safely ordered as pleasant tonics when the appetite is fitful and delicate . . ." (p. 1002)

1881

Pavy, F. W. A TREATISE ON FOOD AND DIETETICS. PHYSIOLOGI-CALLY AND THERAPEUTICALLY CONSIDERED. *New York: William Wood & Company, Second edition. (First edition, 1874)*

Written by a physician and lecturer on physiology, this book deals mainly with food, alimentary principles, principles of dietetics, therapeutic dietetics, and hospital dietaries. One section is devoted to wine, its chemistry and its physiologic effects. On appetite he comments: "They [German wines] are of light alcoholic strength, and are characterized by their marked and peculiar aroma or fragrance, and their acidulous nature. These properties render them . . . an excitant of the appetite." (p. 261)

1891–1894

Charcot, J. M.; Bouchard and Brissaud TRAITE DE MEDECINE. *Paris: G. Masson, 6 vols.*

A classic handbook on medicine compiled by the famous neurologist Charcot. The third volume of this series deals with diseases of the buccal cavity, of the pharynx and adjoining organs, of the stomach, pancreas, intestines, peritoneum and biliary ducts. On stomatitis, Charcot states: "The patient should be nourished with soft boiled eggs, milk, bouillon . . . and in addition generous wines." (Vol. 3, p. 17)

1916
Carlson, Anton Julius: THE CONTROL OF HUNGER IN HEALTH
AND DISEASE. *The University of Chicago Press.*

A classic study on the mechanism and control of hunger
and appetite. The work discusses the relation of hunger to
appetite, hunger and disease, control of the hunger mechanism
and the secretion of "appetite" juice in man. "Wine, beer,
brandy and pure alcohol (diluted) introduced directly into
the stomach, inhibit the hunger contractions and the tonus
of the empty stomach instead of increasing them . . . Alcoholic beverages can therefore not initiate or increase hunger
. . . Since most of the alcoholic beverages stimulate the end-
organs of taste and smell as well as those of general sensibility
in the mouth cavity and in the esophagus, it is possible that
this stimulation in some way augments or initiates *appetite*
for food. If this is the case, we have the singular condition of
alcoholic beverages augmenting appetite and inhibiting hunger at the same time. There can be little doubt that cerebral
states, as modified by training or habit, are also factors in
this apparent action of alcoholic beverages on appetite." (pp.
178–180)

1917
Labbé, Marcel REGIMES ALIMENTAIRES. *Paris: J. B. Baillière
et fils., Second edition. (First edition, 1910)*

A handbook giving dietetic advice and diets for various
diseases, and showing discretion in the recommendation of
wine. "A little wine or a few drops of cognac in milk are
usually well tolerated and sustain the strength of the subject
in affections of the esophagus." (p. 415)

1925
Lee, R. I. THE USE OF ALCOHOL IN MEDICAL PRACTICE.
J.A.M.A., 85:577–579.

A paper read before the Section on Pharmacology and
Therapeutics at an AMA meeting, in which the author gives
his views on the clinical uses of alcohol. It is the belief of
the author that the main benefit of alcohol is to be attributed
to its pharmacologic effect in the production of euphoria, and
that—in the strict sense—indications for the clinical use of
alcohol are very rare. In a discussion of the paper, Dr. A. E.
Roussel comments: ". . . certain it is that when strychnin and
bitter tonics are often without immediate result in the production of an appetite and in improvement of digestion, a

good Burgundy wine will effect the results we are seeking to obtain." (p. 579)

1933
Malachowski, T. VIN ET L'APPETIT. *J. Méd. Bordeaux, 110:732.*
An article championing the use of wine in anorexia, and in which the author states: "Wine has the advantage over milk of being able to stimulate and maintain the appetite."

1950
Reich, Philipp WEIN-KOMPENDIUM FÜR DEN ARZT. ÜEBERBLICK UND WEGWEISER. *Stuttgart: Wissenschaftliche Verlagsgesellschaft.*
"There is no drug which can replace wine, particularly in the constant fight against loss of appetite . . . In instances of anorexia, one-half glass or more of wine taken one-half hour before mealtime is a proved remedy." (pp. 124, 140)

1957
Lefft, H. H. SOME NUTRITIONAL AND THERAPEUTIC ASPECTS OF WINE AND COGNAC. *Int. Rec. Med., 170:361–368.*
An article reviewing the effects of beverage alcohol on the digestive and cardiovascular systems, in which the therapeutic uses of wine and brandy in a number of conditions are discussed. Referable to appetite, the author states: "Beverage alcohol in moderate quantities is an unparalleled stimulator of appetite. It impels increased flow of saliva and gastric juice and reduces consciousness of psychic factors that can contribute to anorexia." (p. 363)

CONTRAINDICATIONS

While there are no reports on clinical or laboratory experiments to indicate that wine is contraindicated in esophageal and pharyngeal pathology, common sense provides adequate authority that it should be avoided in esophagitis, or ulcer, or if it causes discomfort.

3   The Effects of Wine and its Constituents on the Functions and Disorders of the Stomach

EFFECTS ON NORMAL FUNCTIONS

The stomach may be compared to a distensible sac which lies like a closed hammock between the lower end of the esophagus and the jejunal segment of the small bowel. Its muscular wall is thick and capable of powerful and firm contractions. The interior surface of the wall is lined by a delicate membrane in which a variety of cells are embedded, some secreting hydrochloric acid, others basic mucin which acts to protect the gastric wall from auto-digestion, and other cells which secrete digestive enzymes.

The major efforts of digestion occur in the stomach. The partially digested food releases substances which reflexly stimulate the outpouring of secretions from the various cells and organs making up the digestive complex. The churning and constrictive activity of the stomach wall initiates rhythmic constrictions which assist in softening the food and propelling it into the lower segments where it is subjected to the activity of the digestive secretions—acids and enzymes. If too much acid has been secreted, it is neutralized by mucin. When an optimum acid balance is achieved, the action of salivary ptyalin ceases; however, digestion by means of gastric enzymes is continued: pepsin converting protein into proteoses and peptones; renin curdling milk; and lipase initiating the digestion of fats which will be completed in the intestine. The food leaves the stomach in liquid form, as chyme, and enters the intestine where further absorption takes place.

It is recorded that wine stimulates the production of gastric secretions, and enhances the motility of the stomach. Beverages containing 20 per cent or more of alcohol inhibit gastric motility and irritate the mucosa. Occasionally, the action of the secretory cells is paralyzed.

A number of investigators have demonstrated that wine increases the flow of enzymes as well as that of hydrochloric acid, and Ogden (1946) has shown that this effect of wine is independent of its content of alcohol. It has also been demonstrated that the tartrates, phosphates and other constituents of wine act as buffers and perpetuate the flow of gastric juice over extended periods of time. Studies concerning the effect of wine as a tension-reducing agent would indicate its potential use as a prophylactic against dyspepsia—a common disorder of modern man.

1568
Turner, William A BOOK OF WINES . . . *New York: Scholars' Facsimiles and Reprints, 1941.*

". . . wines that are thin and waterish, and gently binding, are not only not noisome unto the head but oft times take away light headaches which come from humours gathered together in the stomach [Galen] . . . white wine is thin, and good for the stomach, and is easily conveyed into the members [Dioscorides] . . . it strengtheneth the stomach [Galen]." (pp. 15, 24–25)

1825
Magendie, F. PRECIS ELEMENTAIRE DE PHYSIOLOGIE. *Paris: Mequignon-Marvis, 2 vols., Second edition. (First edition, 1816–1817)*

A comprehensive study of human physiology by an outstanding scientist of the 19th century. In a section devoted to the effects of liquids on digestion, Magendie states: ". . . liquids facilitate the digestion of solid foods; probably this is produced in a variety of ways. Watery liquids soften the food, even dissolving some of them; in this way chymification and the passage of foods through the pylorus is aided. Wine serves analogous functions, but only for substances which it is capable of dissolving; furthermore, it excites the mucous membrane of the stomach, by direct contact, and causes an increased secretion of gastric juice." (Vol. 2, p. 145)

1856
Moleschott, Jacob, and J. Scoffern THE CHEMISTRY OF FOOD
AND DIET; WITH A CHAPTER ON FOOD ADULTERATIONS. THE
TREATISE ON FOOD AND DIET BEING A TRANSLATION OF LEHRE
DER NAHRUNGSMITTEL FÜR DAS VOLK, BY PROFESSOR MOLE-
SCHOTT, OF ZÜRICH, BY EDWARD BRONNER. THE CHAPTER ON
FOOD ADULTERATIONS BY JOHN SCOFFERN. *London: Houlston
and Stoneman.*

"Wine . . . if moderately taken stimulates the different digestive glands to an abundant secretion and therefore promotes digestion." (p. 80)

1864
Sheen, James Richmond WINES AND OTHER FERMENTED
LIQUORS; FROM THE EARLIEST AGES TO THE PRESENT TIME.
DEDICATED TO ALL CONSUMERS IN THE UNITED KINGDOM.
London: Robert Hardwicke.

An extensive discussion on the wines of the world, touching on a variety of subjects, both historical and technical.
Chapter VIII is devoted to the use of wine in health and disease. Referable to "wines containing malic acid, when the
fermentation has been imperfect, the fermentative state of
the liquor is recommenced in the stomach, and carbonic and
other gases are evolved, which distending that organ, oppress
the individual." But, wines "pure in quality and of proper
age, . . . may be said to promote digestion [and] exhilarate
the spirits . . ." (pp. 38–39)

1873
Lankester, E. ON FOOD. BEING LECTURES DELIVERED AT THE
SOUTH KENSINGTON MUSEUM. *London: Robert Hardwicke.*

"In cases where the nervous power of the stomach is feeble,
and the glandular apparatus not performing its duty . . . alcohol, by its action on the nerve of the part, at once . . . brings
the flagging organ up to its duty. It is in this way that it acts
beneficially in many forms of indigestion arising from want of
power in the stomach. It is in this way, too, that it acts beneficially in . . . individuals whose minds are intensely engaged,
and in whom the whole nervous energy of the body seems
concentrated in the brainwork that is going on. Alcohol, in the
form of wine or beer, seems to make that impression on the
stomach which calls the nervous energy from the remoter
organ and concentrates it upon the important work that is
going on in the stomach . . . Sparkling or effervescing wines

are agreeable to the palate, and, . . . they sometimes appear to assist in the digestion of the food with which they are taken. In some cases, however, there can be no doubt that they produce injury. When new, they communicate the state of change in which they are to the contents of the stomach, and [thereby] interfere with the healthy process of digestion. They are less liable to disagree when they are dry and contain but little sugar." (pp. 199, 239–240)

1882
Buchner, W. EIN BEITRAG ZUR LEHRE VON DER EINWIRKUNG DES ALKOHOLS AUF DIE MAGENVERDAUUNG. *Deutsch. Arch. Klin. Med., 29:537–554.*

A report on successive series of similar experiments carried out on: a) normal adult males, b) adult female patients, and c) on artificial digestion. All the subjects received a carefully controlled diet to which wine, beer and/or alcohol was added on alternate days. In the experiments on artificial digestion, alcohol was added to the digestive surrogate. The results of the experiments on artificial digestion showed that: 1) when a 10% solution of alcohol was added to an artificial surrogate, it did not influence the rate of digestion of a piece of meat suspended in the medium; 2) a 20% solution of alcohol retarded digestion; and 3) at higher concentrations of alcohol digestion was completely inhibited; 4) undiluted beer inhibited artificial digestion completely and dilutions of beer with water retarded digestion; 5) red and sweet wines followed the pattern established for beer, but white wines retarded digestion exclusively, regardless of their alcohol concentration.

The series of experiments on human subjects showed that: 1) beer and wine, even in very small amounts, when added to the diet of healthy subjects, seem to have an undesirable effect on digestion; and 2) in human subjects suffering from disturbances in resorption or secretion, both beer and wine were shown to cause complete inhibition of digestion.

1884
Jaillet, Jules DE L'ALCOOL, SA COMBUSTION, SON ACTION PHYSI-OLOGIQUE, SON ANTIDOTE. *Paris: O. Doin.*

An objective appraisal of the physiologic effects of alcohol and alcoholic beverages. "Ingested in very moderate quantities, in the form of wine, beer, spirits and even whiskey, when the stomach is full, alcohol favors digestion by augmenting the gastric secretion . . . To obtain these effects, the advantageous dose ought not to exceed 50 cc. in 48 hours; this dose, in the form of wine, should be taken with the meals." (p. 82)

1885

Schellhaas, H. BEITRÄGE ZUR PATHOLOGIE DES MAGENS. *Deutsch. Arch. Klin. Med., 36:427–453.*

Experiments concerning the effects of alcohol on gastric digestion in adult human patients, in artificial digestion, and studies on the acidity of the gastric juice, are reported. The following tests were used to measure free hydrochloric acid: methyl-aniline-violet, Tropacolin, and ferric chloride-carbolic acid. Solutions of alcohol and undiluted wine were used as the test liquid. When free hydrochloric acid was present either in the stomach or in the digestive surrogate, retardation of digestion occurred when the concentration of alcohol reached 10 per cent. In the presence of gastric carcinoma, even minimal amounts of alcohol completely inhibit digestion.

1886

Caillol de Poncy, O. ACTION DU ROUGE DE BORDEAUX SUR LA DIGESTION. *Marseille Méd., 23:194–199.*

Experiments to determine the effect of red Bordeaux wine on digestion are described. Animals (cats and guinea pigs) were used. The results indicated that the digestion of starch was not affected, but the digestion of proteins was retarded.

Roberts, Sir William LECTURES ON DIETETICS AND DYSPEPSIA . . . *London: Smith, Elder & Co., Second edition.*

"As used dietetically, sherry must figure as having frequently an important retarding effect on peptic digestion . . . This wine is used with dinner by some persons very freely . . . In the more common practice of taking two or three wine-glasses of sherry with dinner, we see probably a double action—a stimulating action on the secretion of gastric juice, and on the muscular contractions of the stomach, and a slight retarding effect on the speed of the chemical process . . . In smaller proportions, a wine glass or so, sherry would act as a pure stimulant to digestion . . . The more sparing use of these wines [hock, claret, and champagne], a glass or two, with dinner or luncheon would evidently not produce any appreciable retardation of peptic action, but would, like corresponding doses of sherry, act as pure stimulants . . . With large quantities we may obtain retardation, with small quantities we may obtain acceleration of gastric digestion." (pp. 42–44)

1898
Chittenden, R. H.; L. B. Mendel, and H. C. Jackson A FURTHER
STUDY OF THE INFLUENCE OF ALCOHOL AND ALCOHOLIC DRINKS
UPON DIGESTION, WITH SPECIAL REFERENCE TO SECRETION.
Amer. J. Physiol., 1:164–209.

"Upon gastric secretion, alcohol and alcoholic fluids have a
marked effect, increasing very greatly both the flow of gastric
juice and also its content of acid and total solids . . . it is seen
that side by side with the greater or lesser retardation of digestive proteolysis caused by alcoholic beverages there occurs
an increased flow of gastric juice rich in acid and of unquestionable digestive power . . . Since, however, the stimulation
of gastric secretion induced by alcohol is brought about . . .
also by the indirect action of alcohol absorbed from the intestine, it follows that possible inhibition would probably be
of shorter duration than the stimulation of secretion, . . ."
(pp. 207–208)

1903
Billings, John S. PHYSIOLOGICAL ASPECTS OF THE LIQUOR PROB-
LEM. *Boston and New York: Houghton, Mifflin and Company,
2 vols.*

"The data obtained . . . tend to show that when alcohol and
alcoholic fluids are taken into the stomach there is a marked
increase in the flow of gastric juice accompanied by an increase in the content of the essential constituents, pepsin and
hydrochloric acid, as well as in the content of total solid matter . . . Whiskey, brandy, sherry, claret, beer and porter, as
well as pure alcohol, all agree in producing direct and indirect stimulation of gastric secretion, increasing both the rate
of flow of the gastric juice and the concentration of the fluid
. . . Not until the digestive mixture contains five to ten per
cent of absolute alcohol is the action of the gastric juice materially interfered with. With these proportions of absolute alcohol, equal to ten or twenty per cent of proof spirit, retardation of proteolysis becomes noticeable . . . In considering the
influence of wines upon the solvent action of the gastric juice
. . . sherry wine . . . containing from twenty to twenty-one per
cent of alcohol . . . [causes] marked retardation of gastric proteolysis. The inhibition produced is out of all proportion to
the amount of alcohol present . . . The retarding action of
sherry is due, mainly at least, to the solid matters present in
the wine . . . With clarets, on the other hand, containing approximately ten per cent of alcohol, small amounts (say one

per cent) added to gastric juice lead to an increase in the rate of digestion . . . In view of what has been stated regarding the rapid withdrawal of alcohol from the stomach by absorption, together with the action of the absorbed alcohol upon secretion, it would appear that the stimulating effect of alcoholic fluids upon gastric secretion would be far more lasting than the inhibitory action upon the chemical process of digestion, and thus lead to a marked increase in the rate of digestion." (Vol. I, pp. 143–144, 146–148, 151)

Cabot, R. C. STUDIES ON THE ACTION OF ALCOHOL IN DISEASE, ESPECIALLY UPON THE CIRCULATION. *Boston Med. Surg. J., 149:93–101.*

A brief review of the data concerning alcohol and its physiologic effects on the organ systems of the human body. In the section on alcohol and digestion, the author states: "After absorption [either from the stomach or from the intestines] alcohol acts upon the stomach through the nervous system, and exerts a favorable influence both on its secretion and on its motility. But the nervous system is soon blunted to its influence, so that more and more is needed to influence digestion." (p. 94)

1905
Triboulet, H. Felix Mathieu, and Roger Minot TRAITE D'ALCOOLISME. *Preface by Prof. Joffroy. Paris: Masson et Cie.*

A treatise on alcoholism written for the physician. In the section on the physiologic effects of alcohol, it is stated: "In small doses, alcohol excites the function of the stomach mucosa and definitely increases gastric secretion: however, this is a reaction common to any other excitants." (p. 94)

1907
Commission on Light Wines A SPECIAL REPORT ON THEIR CHEMICAL COMPOSITION AND DIETETIC VALUE. *The Hospital, 42:284–295.*

A report on experimental (in vitro) findings with regard to the physiologic effects of wine. The results indicated that up to a 3% concentration of alcohol in the stomach had an obviously stimulating influence on the chemical process of digestion. (Ten oz. of wine taken during a meal did not exceed a concentration of 2% of alcohol in the stomach.)

1910
McBride, C. A. THE MODERN TREATMENT OF ALCOHOLISM AND

DRUG NARCOTISM. *New York: Rebman Company.*

A book in which a physician who specialized in the treatment of "alcohol and drug inebriates" records his experiences and methods. He discusses inebriety, its causes and forms, pathologic changes due to alcohol, and methods of treatment. "If given in large quantities and concentrated, it [alcohol] diminishes the amount of gastric and pancreatic secretions; but if given in small quantities and well diluted, it is said to increase the flow of secretions. In large quantities alcohol has a distinctly retarding effect on the activity of the salivary, gastric, and pancreatic ferments . . . So far as the gastric secretion is concerned, it is thought by some that this retardation is due to the precipitation of the pepsin." (pp. 21–22)

1911

Saltykow, S. EXPERIMENTELLE FORSCHUNG ÜBER DIE PATHOLOGISCHE ANATOMIE DES ALKOHOLISMUS CHRONICUS. *Zbl. Allg. Path. Anat., 22:849–880.*

A study of the biologic changes resulting from chronic alcoholism. A state of chronic alcoholism was induced in experimental animal and tissues and organ changes, after sacrifice, were observed. "This study demonstrated the appearance of catarrhal changes of the stomach mucosa; however, one should keep in mind that these changes are not specific to alcohol alone and can be induced by a number of other substances which irritate the stomach." (p. 872)

Watson, Chalmers FOOD AND FEEDING IN HEALTH AND DISEASE. A MANUAL OF PRACTICAL DIETETICS. *New York: William Wood & Company.*

Written by the editor of *The Encyclopedia Medica,* this book treats in great detail the problems which a student of dietetics might encounter. It discusses first the physiological aspects of digestion, and then a great variety of foods and beverages. The book also considers food for the various age-levels, for the patient in the hospital and at home, and diets for diseases of almost all systems and organs. "The chief effect of alcohol when taken in small doses is to increase the motility of the stomach, and thus indirectly stimulate digestion." (p. 143)

1914

Babkin, B. P. DIE ÄUSSERE SEKRETION DER VERDAUUNGSDRÜSEN. *Berlin: Julius Springer Verlag.*

One of the earliest definitive works on the secretion of the

digestive glands, reprinted into many editions, the latest in
English in 1950. The author, a student and collaborator of I.
V. Pavlov, discusses all of the secretory glands of the gastrointestinal tract, the functional role of bile, and certain motor
appearances of the digestive canal. Regarding the effect of
alcohol on gastric secretion, the author states that it markedly
stimulates such secretion in solutions as low as 6% and that
a 10% solution of alcohol in distilled water almost doubles
the output of gastric secretion high in digestive power; but
alcohol in concentrations above 10% has an inhibiting effect
on gastric secretions.

1921

Haneborg, A. THE EFFECTS OF ALCOHOL ON DIGESTION IN THE
STOMACH. *Acta Med. Scand. (Suppl.), 55:1–124.*

To 92 human subjects test meals, with ethyl alcohol, cognac, aquavit, claret, rhine wine, and beer, were administered.
The stomach contents were then periodically recovered by
esophageal tube. Haneborg found that wines and beers at
first slowed proteolysis and then, over a period of hours,
gradually and markedly increased it.

Mallory, W. J. EFFECT OF ALCOHOL ON THE GASTROINTESTINAL
TRACT. *Med. Red., 100:275–277.*

"In conditions of hypermotility of the stomach . . . alcoholic beverages . . . act both locally and after absorption on
the mechanism involved;" (p. 277)

1923

Starling, Ernest H. THE ACTION OF ALCOHOL ON MAN . . . *London: Longmans, Green and Co.*

"If alcoholic fluids are introduced into the stomach there
is a rapid secretion of an active gastric juice rich in hydrochloric acid . . . But there is no question that in moderate concentrations . . . alcohol acts as a direct stimulant to gastric
secretion." (p. 110)

1924

Edkins, N., and M. M. Murray INFLUENCE OF CARBON DIOXIDE
ON THE ABSORPTION OF ALCOHOL BY THE GASTRIC MUCOSA. *J.
Physiol., 59:271–275.*

Report of experiments on decerebrated cats in which the

stomach pathway was severed at the esophagus and a cannula inserted into the pylorus. Sixty cc. of 5% alcohol were injected into the pylorus through the cannula and an hour later gastric content was collected and the amount of alcohol determined. It was found that absorption was increased considerably by the simultaneous administration of carbon dioxide and alcohol.

1925

Simici, D., Voiculesco, E. and G. Vajez CONTRIBUTIONS EXPERIMENTALES CONCERNANT L'ACTION DE L'ALCOOL SUR LA SECRETION ET L'EVACUATION DE L'ESTOMAC.*Bull. & Mém. Soc. Méd. Hôp. Bucharest, 7:139–146.*

1928

Farrell, J. I. CONTRIBUTIONS TO THE PHYSIOLOGY OF GASTRIC SECRETION. XIII: THE RESPONSE OF THE GLANDS TO SUBSTANCES APPLIED TO THE GASTRIC MUCOSA. *Amer. J. Physiol., 85:672–684.*

A report on experiments carried out at the Department of Physiology, Northwestern University Medical School, with the purpose of determining the chemical action of various substances on the gastric mucosa. The subjects were dogs, and the substances used were: water, hydrochloric acid, sodium bicarbonate, lactic acid, alcohol, bitter tonics, meat and meat products, egg white, milk and milk products, sucrose, fat and fatty acids, coffee, and mustard oil. With regard to alcohol, the results showed that, "Alcohol [10% solution] in moderate quantities stimulates gastric secretion by local contact with the gastric mucosa." (p. 683)

Franzen, G. UNTERSUCHUNGEN ÜBER ALKOHOL. VII. ALKOHOLWIRKUNGEN AUF DIE MAGENVERDAUUNG. *Arch. Exp. Path. Pharm., 134:129–141.*

A report on experimental studies, carried out at the Institute of Pharmacology of the University of Jena, designed to demonstrate the action of alcohol on gastric digestion. The experiments were carried out on normal human subjects and also in the absence of artificial digestion. It was found that "certain concentrations of alcohol have a beneficial effect on artificial as well as natural pepsin digestion. Alcohol in concentrations of 5–7% and over has a retarding effect on the emptying mechanism of the stomach; in lower concentrations it is without effect or is slightly stimulating to the action of the stomach." (p. 141)

1929
Decref, J. LE VIN ET SA VALEUR ALIMENTAIRE ET HYGIENIQUE. *Rapports Comites Nat. Scient. Off. Int. Vin, pp. 1–6.*
"Pure wine, such as is produced in Spain, drunk in moderate quantity, is not only a hygienic beverage, but also stimulates the gastric secretions." (p. 5)

Petrovitch, A., and E. Bokanova L'ACTION DE L'ALCOOL SUR LE CHIMISME GASTRIQUE. *C. R. Soc. Biol., 102:633.*
A short report on experimental work at the University of Smolensk. The action of alcohol on gastric chemistry, after oral and intravenous administration, was measured in human subjects. A 15% solution of alcohol was used as the test solution and gastric contents collected by duodenal tube. The results indicated that alcohol acts directly on the stomach mucosa and elicits increased gastric secretion.

1930
Gukasian, A. G. EFFECTS OF ALCOHOL AND BEER ON SECRETORY FUNCTIONS OF THE STOMACH. *Russ. klin., 13:659–674.*
The author, a member of the Therapeutic Clinic of Moscow, describes experiments in which the effects of beer and alcohol on gastric secretion were observed. From these studies, the author concludes that alcohol, especially when using a 10% solution, markedly stimulates secretion. The author suggests that alcohol solutions not be used for the examination of gastric secretion, since even weak solutions of alcohol can damage the mucous membrane.

1931
Dunn, F. L., and A. M. Perley INFLUENCE OF ETHYL ALCOHOL UPON GASTRIC ABSORPTION OF PHENOL IN RABBITS. *J. Lab. Clin. Med., 16:1066–1068.*
Report of experimental studies on rabbits receiving oral solutions of phenol, and phenol plus alcohol. Blood samples were taken at varying intervals by heart puncture. The group receiving the phenol plus alcohol mixture showed a slightly more rapid rise in free blood phenol, but final levels in the two groups were essentially the same. "The effect of alcohol on gastric absorption of phenol is slight and the *apparent* in-

crease in toxicity is probably due to a superadded alcohol poisoning." (p. 1068)

Gradinesco, A., and H. Palmhert INFLUENCE DES ALCOOLS ETHYLIQUE ET METHYLIQUE SUR LA DIGESTION DU SUC GASTRIQUE ARTIFICIEL ET NATUREL. *J. Physiol. Path. Gen., 29:45–51.*

The effect of ethyl and methyl alcohol on natural and artificial digestion was studied. The authors found that artificial and natural gastric juices give concordant results; that both methyl and ethyl alcohol inhibit the digestion of solid protein matter, and that ethyl alcohol has a more pronounced effect than methyl.

1932

Newman, H. W., and H. G. Mehrtens EFFECT OF INTRAVENOUS INJECTION OF ETHYL ALCOHOL ON GASTRIC SECRETION IN MAN. *Proc. Soc. Exp. Biol. Med., 30:145–148.*

A report on experiments designed to show whether intravenous alcohol is as active a stimulant of gastric secretion as alcohol administered orally. The tests were carried out on human subjects, using a 25% ethyl alcohol solution in normal saline, injected intravenously at a constant rate of 10 cc. per minute. It was found that "alcohol intravenously in man produces an increase in gastric acidity . . . it would seem possible that the seat of action of alcohol as a stimulus to gastric secretion lies neither in the general circulation, nor at the surface of the gastric mucosa, but somewhere between the two." (pp. 147–148)

Streicher, M. H. GASTRIC ACHYLIA: GASTRIC ACIDITY STUDIES WITH HISTAMINE AND SEVEN PER CENT ALCOHOL. *J.A.M.A., 99:1745–1746.*

A brief report on experimental work which indicated that 0.01 mg. of histamine per kilogram of body weight markedly stimulates gastric acidity. In 40% of the subjects the same result was obtained with 8 oz. of a 7% alcohol solution. The author suggests discontinuing the diagnostic use of histamine and replacing it with alcohol.

1934

Bravo, J. EFFETS DU VIN DANS LES PROCESSUS DIGESTIFS. *IIe Congrès Nat'l. Méd. Amis des Vins de France, Béziers, pp. 297–301.*

"Wine taken in moderate quantities . . . stimulates gastric

digestion but only when the concentration of alcohol in the stomach does not exceed 10% . . . The quantity of wine injested should never exceed 1 to 1.2 gr. of alcohol per kilogram of body weight." (pp. 299–301)

Brüll, Z., and E. Froehlich BIETRÄGE ZUM MECHANISMUS DER MAGENSAFTSEKRETION. I. DIE MAGENSAFTSEKRETION NACH PARENTERALER UND STOMACHALER ZUFUHR VON AETHYLALKOHOL UND KOFFEIN. *Arch. Verdauungskr. 56:71–80.*

Report of experiments, carried out at the medical clinic of the University of Prague, in which gastric secretion, after parenteral administration of ethyl alcohol and coffee, was measured. It was found that 20 cc. of a 15% solution of alcohol administered perorally had less effect on the gastric secretion than the same amount administered intravenously.

Caujolle, F. INFLUENCE DU VIN SUR L'ACTIVITE DES FERMENTS DIGESTIFS IN VITRO. *IIe Congrès Nat'l. Méd. Amis des Vins de France, Béziers, pp. 175–178.*

A preliminary report on studies carried out at the Medical and Pharmaceutical Laboratories of the University of Toulouse. The effect of wine on the digestive enzymes was studied in vitro in a series of 24 tests. The results, thus far, showed that amylolysis is influenced by the acidity of wine in that a decrease of lysis occurs; pepsin proteolysis, however, requiring an acid milieu, was stimulated by the acidity of wine.

Harmon, P. H., and E. Andrews EFFECT OF HISTAMINE AND ALCOHOL ON ACID SECRETION OF STOMACH OF POST-OPERATIVE CASES. *Proc. Soc. Exp. Biol. Med., 32:39–40.*

Report of an experimental study on human post-operative subjects using histamine (0.5 or 1.0 mg. by hypodermic) and alcohol (50 cc. Sauternes—15% alcohol—by nasal tube) to provoke gastric secretion. It was found that "histamine and alcohol have their usual action of stimulating gastric secretion in the postoperative surgical patient. Their administration is clinically beneficial." (p. 40)

Von Friedrich, L., and G. A. Bokor DIE WIRKUNG DES REINEN ALKOHOLS AUF DIE MAGENMOTILITÄT. *Arch. Verdauungskr., 55: 202–212.*

Experiments on human subjects showed that 300 ml. of 5–10 per cent alcohol solution taken with or after a standard opaque meal, slightly delayed the emptying time of the stomach. There was, however, some increase in peristalsis.

1936

Barlow, O. W. STUDIES ON THE PHARMACOLOGY OF ETHYL ALCOHOL. I. A COMPARATIVE STUDY OF PHARMACOLOGIC EFFECTS OF GRAIN AND SYNTHETIC ETHYL ALCOHOLS. II. A CORRELATION OF THE LOCAL IRRITANT, ANESTHETIC AND TOXIC EFFECTS OF THREE POTABLE WHISKEYS WITH THEIR ALCOHOLIC CONTENT. *J. Pharmacol. Exp. Therap., 56:117–146.*

In this study, the effect of grain ethyl alcohol on the gastrointestinal tract was compared to that of synthetic ethyl alcohol and to various blended whiskeys. Twelve adult males received 50 cc. of a 7% solution of alcohol from each fluid tested (3 types of blended whiskey, grain and synthetic ethyl alcohol); several days later, the same subjects received 50 cc. of a 30% solution of alcohol made from the same liquids. The stomach contents were examined under fasting conditions, and at intervals during a 90-minute period following administration of test fluids. The effects of synthetic alcohol did not differ from grain alcohol or blended whiskey. The solution of 30% alcohol produced a greater stimulation of secretion than that produced by the 7% solution, but the 30% solution was definitely more irritating to the mucous membranes of the stomach.

Blotner, H. EFFECT OF ALCOHOL ON DIGESTION BY GASTRIC JUICE, TRYPSIN, AND PANCREATIN. *J.A.M.A., 106:1970–1971.*

Experimental studies on artificial digestion and human subjects carried out at the Peter Bent Brigham Hospitals, Medical Clinic. The results showed that a given "amount of alcohol destroys the proteolytic activity of certain gastrointestinal enzymes in vitro and in vivo." (p. 1971)

1937

Krueger, L., and F. C. MacIntosh ALCOHOL AS A STOMACHIC. *Amer. J. Dig. Dis., 4:104–107.*

Report on experimental studies on dogs in which the authors "have been able to show that alcohol, besides stimulating the secretion of fluid and acid by the stomach, may, in certain circumstances, stimulate also the secretion of pepsin. The necessary condition for this additional action is that the alcohol should be relished. It then becomes a positive condition stimulus for gastric secretion, increasing the output of pepsin reflexly through activation of the vagal secretory centers." (p. 104)

Weissenbach, R. J., and G. Faroy LE VIN ET LE JUS DE RAISIN DANS LA DIÉTÉTIQUE ET LE TRAITEMENT DES AFFECTIONS GAS-TRO-INTÉSTINALES. *IVe Congrès Nat'l. Méd. Amis des Vins de France, Alger. pp. 86–158.*

"The alcohol, sugars, acids and vitamins in wine excite gastric secretion which is rich in chlorhydric acid and pepsin . . . During digestion of foods wine helps maintain a favorable pH milieu in the stomach." (pp. 101–102)

1940

Beckers, R. THE NUTRITIVE VALUE OF WINE. *Wines & Vines, 21:14, 26.*

"Through its components, wine releases and excites the gastric juices. It gives to the region of the stomach, conditions favorable to digestion." (p. 14)

Dybing, O., and E. W. Rasmussen DIE RESORPTION DES ATHYL-ALKOHOLS AUS DEM MAGEN UND DARM DER RATTE. *Biochem. Z., 306:337–342.*

A report of experimental studies from the Institute of Pharmacology of the University of Oslo. Male white rats received 5, 10, 20 and 40% solutions of alcohol (intraperitoneally and perorally) after a 36-hour period of starvation during which time they had access to fluids. It was found that in the rat, resorption of the lower concentrations of alcohol occurred from the stomach, but that blood levels corresponding to the higher concentrations of alcohol were found after resorption from the intestines.

Engler, G. A. HEALTH VALUES OF CHAMPAGNE. *Wines & Vines, 21:5.*

"Champagne is a tonic for the stomach; . . . [it] helps to make better use of the normal diet."

Gray, J. S., and W. H. Bachrach EFFECTS OF ATROPINE AND FAT ON GASTRIC SECRETION STIMULATED BY ALCOHOL. *Proc. Soc. Exp. Biol. Med., 43:36–38.*

Report on experiments carried out at the Northwestern University Medical School, Department of Physiology. These tests were designed to investigate the mode of action of the alcohol test meal and the possible influence of other drugs on its action. Dogs with Pavlov-type gastric pouches were used and the test meals consisted of ground beef hearts boiled in water alone, in water plus olive oil, and in water plus atropine sulfate; in the second series the meat meals were replaced by 120 cc. of a 7% solution of alcohol administered by stomach tube. The results showed that "1 mg. of atropine sulfate completely abolished the gastric secretory response to the meat meal, but only partially reduced the response to 7% alcohol. Similarly, the alcohol stimulus proved to be more resistant than the meat meal to the inhibitory action of olive oil." (p. 38) The suggestion is made that the action of alcohol on the gastric glands is similar to that of histamine.

Lacroix, P. LE VIN. *Concours Méd., 62:967–969.*
"Wine especially should be taken in small doses and, generally, with the meal when the absorption of liquids from the stomach is retarded." (p. 969)

McGuigan, Hugh Alister APPLIED PHARMACOLOGY. *St. Louis: The C. V. Mosby Company.*
"The effect of alcoholic drinks upon digestion is of great practical importance . . . If they contain substances which have an agreeable taste, they stimulate the psychic secretion of gastric juice . . . Alcohol by direct stimulation of the secretory glands of the stomach can rapidly induce secretion when psychic secretion is absent . . . It has been demonstrated that alcohol also increases the absorption of fluids from the stomach and bowel." (p. 260)

Tudoranu, G.; C. C. Dimitriu, and M. Filipesco INFLUENCE DE L'ABSORPTION GASTRIQUE DE QUELQUES SUBSTANCES SUR LA MOTILITE STOMACALE (VISCEROGRAPHIE). *Bull. Acad. Méd. Roumanie, 5:61–67.*
A series of investigations on human subjects in which 8 different substances were used (alcohol, coffee, sodium chloride, bouillon, extract of spinach, histamine, and sodium bicarbonate) and gastric motility measured with a kymograph. It was found that alcohol (100 cc. of a 10% solution) injected into the stomach inhibits stomach motility.

1941
Tennent, D. M. THE INFLUENCE OF ALCOHOL ON THE EMPTYING

TIME OF THE STOMACH AND THE ABSORPTION OF GLUCOSE. *Quart. J. Stud. Alc., 2:271–276.*

Report of experimental studies from the Laboratory of Applied Physiology, Yale University. Serial studies were done on rats who received alcohol intraperitoneally—a 50% solution in dosages of 3 mg. (or 1 g/kg. of body weight). Controls received an equivalent volume of distilled water. Glucose, 6 g/kg. of body weight, was administered one hour later by stomach tube. It was found that the absorption of glucose is slowed by mild intoxication and markedly inhibited by severe intoxication. This delay in absorption is ascribed to failure of the stomach to empty because of pylorospasm from alcohol which occurred also when the alcohol was administered intraperitoneally.

1942

Lolli, G., and L. A. Greenberg THE EFFECT OF INSULIN ON THE RATE OF DISAPPEARANCE OF ALCOHOL FROM THE STOMACH *Quart. J. Stud. Alc., 3:92–96.*

A series of experiments carried out at the Laboratory of Applied Physiology, Yale University, is reported. Twenty-five and 50% alcohol was administered to rats with and without two and four units of insulin and the emptying time of the stomach observed. The results showed than when 50% alcohol was given, insulin did not increase the rate of elimination of alcohol from the stomach, probably because of severe pylorospasm; when 25% alcohol was given a rapid disappearance occurred. This disappearance rate was due to an increased rate of emptying of the stomach.

Newman, H., and M. Abramson ABSORPTION OF VARIOUS ALCOHOLIC BEVERAGES. *Science, 96:43–44. (Abstract in: Quart. J. Stud. Alc., 3:308, 1942)*

Two healthy adult males were given 13% alcohol by volume in the form of alcohol, scotch and bourbon whiskies, gin, and wine. Venous blood samples were taken 30 minutes after ingestion was completed. After distilled spirits alcohol concentration in the blood was higher and occurred sooner; when the distilled spirits were buffered to the same pH and buffer capacity as that of wine, absorption of alcohol into the blood was found to be identical with that of wine. The authors concluded that "there can be no doubt that the slower absorption of wine . . . is ascribable to its buffer capacity." (p. 44)

1943
Lolli, G., and M. Rubin ALCOHOL AND THE EMPTYING TIME OF
THE STOMACH. *Quart. J. Stud. Alc., 4:64–67.*

Experimental studies carried out at the Laboratory of Applied Physiology, Yale University, are reported. A 25% solution of alcohol (3 g/kg. of body weight) was administered to
rats 2 hours before the administration of a 25% solution of
glucose (2.5 g/kg. of body weight). The amount of glucose
remaining in the stomach was measured serially 1, 2, and 3
hours after its administration. With the amounts of alcohol
given, the decrease in the rate of gastric emptying was marked
enough to be the factor in causing gastric disturbances associated with acute alcoholic intoxication.

1946
Ogden, E., and F. D. Southard, Jr. THE INFLUENCE OF WINE
ON GASTRIC ACIDITY. *Fed. Proc., 5:77.*

Report of experimental work on human subjects who were
given various test fluids (distilled water, whiskey, table wine,
14% ethanol solution, dealcoholized wine, and a solution of
cream of tartar adjusted to approximately the pH and titrable
acidity of wine). Gastric fluid samples were withdrawn every
20 minutes and free and total acidity titrated. The curves
rose highest and were more prolonged after wine.

1947
Rehm, W. S., and L. E. Hokin THE EFFECT OF PILOCARPINE,
MECHOLYL, ATROPINE AND ALCOHOL ON THE GASTRIC POTEN-
TIAL AND THE SECRETION OF HYDROCHLORIC ACID. *Amer. J.
Physiol., 149:162–176.*

Report on experiments carried out at the University of
Louisville School of Medicine, Department of Physiology,
undertaken in an attempt to find out whether electrical energy
furnishes the energy necessary for the production of the osmo-
tic work involved in the formation of hydrochloric acid by
the stomach. Dogs were used and the substances tested were
those given in the title. It was found that "ethyl alcohol-saline
solutions, applied to the mucosa of the stomach for certain
periods of time, did not under the conditions of the experiment result in the secretion of hydrochloric acid. The potential, [however,] was lowered by this procedure." (p. 175)

Tulin, M.; J. Gutmann, and T. P. Almy THE SECRETION OF GAS-

TRIC MUCIN FOLLOWING AN ALCOHOL MEAL STUDIES ON NOR-
MAL SUBJECTS AND PATIENTS WITH GASTRIC ULCER. *Gastroenterology, 9:191–197.*

Experiments are described in which gastric mucin and acid
secretory responses to an alcohol stimulus were determined in
a group of normal subjects and a group of patients with duodenal ulcer. No significant difference in the concentration and
total mucin in the gastric juice was found. The stimulus used
was 120 cc. of a 14% solution of alcohol.

1952

Bernstein, R. E. THE POTASSIUM, SODIUM, AND CALCIUM CON-
TENT OF GASTRIC JUICE. I. NORMAL VALUES. *J. Lab. Clin. Med.,
40:707–717.*

A report of experimental studies on cations in gastric juice
as indicators of gastric mucosa function and its reaction to
various stimuli. For the purpose of this study, fasting gastric
juice was obtained from 50 healthy male subjects. Flame pho-
tometric as well as chemical analytic methods were used. Histamine, alcohol, and insulin were used as a gastric secretory
stimulant. "Fractional removal of gastric juice after the alcohol stimulus [50 ml. of 7% alcohol followed 1–1½ hours
later by 0.1 mg. histamine per 10 kg. of body weight] indicated an increased secretion of acid to attain maximum acidity
values of 0 to 89 mEq per liter, with concomitant decreases
in sodium, potassium, and calcium values." (p. 711)

1953

Sears, W. G. ALCOHOL, DIETETIC INDISCRETION, AND DYSPEPSIA.
Practitioner, 170:43–50.

An article in which the author reviews some of the historically famous dietetic indiscretions (Henry I, who died of a
surfeit of lampreys in 1135, etc.). He then reviews the effect
of alcohol on the digestive system, the gastric mucous membrane and acute catarrhal gastritis and discusses methods of
treatment for the latter.

1954

Hirschowitz, B. I.; S. W. Hartwell, Jr., and H. M. Pollard THE
ACTION OF ALCOHOL ON GASTRIC FUNCTION. *J. Lab. Clin. Med.,
44:812–813.*

A preliminary report on studies to determine the effects of
oral alcohol on gastric functions. Human subjects were used
and the alcohol was administered orally, subcutaneously, and

intravenously. It was found that alcohol acts peripherally at the synaptic level, rather than by any histamine-like action. Blood and gastric alcohol levels were measured. The peak in the gastric level was not reached until 30 minutes after the administration of alcohol. The authors suggest that this phenomenon seemed to indicate an active excretion of alcohol into the stomach and that it may play a part in the pathogenesis of alcoholic gastritis.

1955

Woodward, E. R.; D. S. Slotten, and V. C. Tillmans MECHANISM OF ALCOHOLIC STIMULATION OF GASTRIC SECRETION. *Proc. Soc. Exp. Biol. Med., 89:428–431.*

Experiments on dogs, carried out at the University of California Medical Center, Los Angeles, intended to determine whether alcohol stimulates gastric secretion by liberating histamine from the tissue. Three series of experiments were carried out and it was concluded that, "Dilute alcohol [solution of 5 or 10 per cent] is a powerful stimulant of the 'gastrin' mechanism of the pyeloric antrum. It appears that in response to ingested alcohol, two-thirds of the gastric juice secreted results from this mechanism." (p. 431)

1956

Hirschowitz, B. I.; H. M. Pollard; S. W. Hartwell, and J. London THE ACTION OF ETHYL ALCOHOL ON GASTRIC ACID SECRETION. *Gastroenterology, 30:244–256.*

Experiments to determine the mechanism of alcohol stimulation of gastric secretion are described. The investigations were carried out on human subjects using physiologic saline as the control solution and 4, 8 or 16% alcohol in physiologic saline as the test solution. It was found that alcohol given intravenously consistently stimulated both acid and volume of gastric secretion, and that it acted centrally, the stimulus being mediated through the vagus nerve.

1957

Woodward, E. R.; C. Robertson; H. D. Ruttenberg, and H. Schapiro ALCOHOL AS A GASTRIC SECRETORY STIMULANT. *Gastroenterology, 32:727–737.*

An investigation undertaken to study the effects of alcohol on the antral hormonal mechanism. Dogs with Heidenhain pouches were used for the studies. The results indicated that alcohol is a powerful stimulant of the antral gastrin mechanism. When administered intravenously alcohol proved to be a strong stimulant of gastric secretion, even in the complete absence of the nervous, antral, and intestinal mechanisms for gastric secretion; and, it was learned that alcohol stimulates the intestinal phase of gastric secretion to a lesser degree than the gastric or antral phase.

1961
Weise, R. E.; H. Schapiro, and E. R. Woodward EFFECT OF PARENTERAL ALCOHOL ON GASTRIC SECRETION. *Surg. Forum, 12: 281–282.*

Report of experiments undertaken to determine the site of action of parenteral alcohol and the possible relationship between blood alcohol levels and gastric secretion. Six dogs with Heidenhain pouches were given 100 cc. of 5% alcohol intravenously and serial blood alcohol levels determined, while gastric secretion was assayed. Another six dogs, on whom control assay of gastric secretion had been done, were divided into three groups: 2 dogs underwent bilateral adrenalectomy, 2 hypophysectomy and 2 pancreatectomy. After recovery they received 100 cc. of 5% alcohol intravenously and studies were done as above. A last group of six dogs underwent isolation of cerebral circulation and gastric secretion responses to 0.1 mg. histamine subcutaneously was measured; they were then infused with 200 cc. of 5% alcohol via the femoral vein. The results of all these studies indicated that "gastric-secretion rose simultaneously with blood alcohol levels; [that] isolation of the circulation of the head . . . showed an abolishment or marked decrease in the gastric secretory response" which, the authors felt, might suggest an involvement of the central nervous system.

1963
Maitrya, B. B. INFLUENCE OF ALCOHOL ON GASTRIC SECRETION. *Ann. Biochem. Exp. Med., 23:539–542.*

Alcohol given intragastrically or intravenously stimulated gastric secretion in dogs. Prior injection of atropine partially reduced the secretion induced by intragastric dosages of alcohol, but completely abolished the secretion induced by intravenous alcohol.

1965
Daves, I. A.; J. H. Miller; C. A. E. Lemmi, and J. C. Thompson MECHANISM AND INHIBITION OF ALCOHOL-STIMULATED GAS-

TRIC SECRETION. *Surg. Forum, 16:305–307.*

Controlled experimental studies on 18 dogs provided with denervated gastric pouches led the authors to conclude that alcohol stimulates gastric secretion both by the release of gastrin and by a direct action of the parietal cell. They found no evidence that histamine is involved in either mechanism.

EFFECTS ON ABNORMAL FUNCTIONS

The stomach is subject to a variety of patho-physiologic changes—the more common afflictions being dyspepsia, gastritis, peptic ulcer, and cancer.

Experimental studies concerning either the effects of wine in the production of disorders of the stomach or the use of wine as a therapeutic adjunct are still quite incomplete; however, there are some studies, primarily clinical reports, which indicate that wine is useful in syndromes in which atony or dyspepsia predominate.

In a study of patients with peptic ulcer, cancer, achylia gastrica, dyspepsia and other gastric disorders, Dr. Frehse (1923) found that: 1) in the presence of ulcer and cancer, alcohol decreased the acidity of the stomach; 2) in achylia gastrica alcohol produced no noticeable effects; and 3) in dyspepsia gastric acidity was increased by the alcohol. Holler and co-workers (1950) found that gastric acidity lagged in normal subjects after the administration of 300 cc. of 5% alcohol by stomach tube.

In general, the consensus is that light wines aid digestion actively, and that red wines are useful in hypochlorhydria. Some authors, especially Italian and French, believe that when malnutrition complicates an existing disorder of digestion, enemata of wine may be helpful.

1821
Philip, A. P. W. A TREATISE ON DIGESTION AND ITS CONSE-QUENCES. *London: T. and G. Underwood. Quoted* BY WILLIAM KITCHINER: THE ART OF INVIGORATING AND PROLONGING LIFE . . . *London: Hurst, Robinson, and Co., Fifth edition. (p. 162)*

"Dyspeptics who have been accustomed to its use, cannot be deprived of it—a very moderate use of wine can hardly be said to be injurious."

1838
Buchan, William DOMESTIC MEDICINE. A TREATISE ON THE PRE-VENTION AND CURE OF DISEASES, BY REGIMEN AND SIMPLE MED-ICINES: WITH DIRECTIONS FOR THE MANAGEMENT OF COMMON CASES IN SURGERY, AS FRACTURES, DISLOCATIONS AND WOUNDS:

THE TREATMENT PECULIAR TO THE DISEASES OF WOMEN AND
CHILDREN: WITH OBSERVATIONS ON THE ART OF PRESERVING
HEALTH, WITHOUT THE AID OF MEDICINE: AND A TREATISE ON
ANIMAL, VEGETABLE, MINERAL AND AERIAL POISONS, POINTING
OUT THE SYMPTOMS, ANTIDOTES AND MEANS OF CURE, IN CASES
OF POISONING . . . REVISED, ENLARGED AND ADAPTED TO THE DIS-
EASES OF THE UNITED STATES. *Cincinnati: U. P. James.*

Compiled by an English physician, this all-encompassing
treatise was intended not only for the general practitioner, but
also for the use of laymen when medical aid was not available.
In the section on "Medicinal Preparations" wine is listed and
described as follows: "The effects of wine are to raise the
pulse, promote perspiration, warm the habit, and exhilarate
the spirits. The red wines, besides these effects, have an astringent quality, by which they strengthen the tone of the stomach and intestines . . ." (p. 701) This is followed by a list
of six medicated wines for use in disorders of the stomach.

1859
Miller, James ALCOHOL: ITS PLACE AND POWER. *(From the 19.
Glasgow edition) Philadelphia: Lindsay & Blakiston.*
The author compiled this monograph at the request of the
Scottish Temperance League which was "anxious to have a
work of high authority on the Medical view of the Temperance
question . . ." In this monograph, the author discusses alcohol
as a poison, as a food, as a medicine and as a luxury. In recounting the effects of alcohol as a medicine, the author states:
"This, too [comparing it to its effect as a poison] is great . . .
[Nonetheless] in dyspeptics of a certain class, in whom the
stomach is deficient in tone and energy, small and cautious
doses of the milder alcoholics—such as wine and malt liquors—may be of service." (pp. 96, 98)

1873
Becquerel, A. TRAITE ELEMENTAIRE D'HYGIENE PRIVEE ET PUB-
LIQUE. *Paris: P. Asselin, Fifth edition. (First edition, Labé,
1851)*
An uncritical treatise in which the medical uses of the various French—and some other—wines are discussed. "Acid
wines of cold climates are bad for the stomach, producing gastric disturbances, dyspepsia, and often diarrhea . . . Bordeaux
wines are slightly tonic; they are suitable in cases of dyspepsia and convalescence." (pp. 684, 686)

1875
Joffroy, A. DE LA MEDICATION PAR L'ALCOOL. *Paris: A. Delahaye.*

"In dispepsia where alcohol is indicated and the stomach cannot tolerate alcoholic drinks, one can use wine enemas, as recommended by Dr. Aran: 150 to 200 gr. of wine to which a few drops of laudanum have been added." (p. 142)

1877
Anstie, Francis E. ON THE USES OF WINES IN HEALTH AND DISEASE. *London: Macmillan and Co.*

"There are, however, a considerable number of cases of dyspepsia, to which there is a tendency, at present, to give the title of catarrhal, simply on the ground that the dyspepsia and want of appetite are accompanied by a certain amount of apparent enlargement of the tongue, and exhaustion of its epithelium, with perhaps a few red points near the tip; but in which the original cause of the mischief is, in truth, nothing but nervous depression. For such cases as these a fixed moderate allowance of a generous wine is very helpful . . . [for such a purpose the wine should be] (a) medium alcoholic strength, and (b) good original vinous flavour; . . . A moderate amount of *astringency* perhaps may increase somewhat the good effects of such wines upon the appetite; . . ." (p. 64)

Trousseau, A. CLINIQUE MEDICALE DE L'HOTEL-DIEU DE PARIS. *Paris: J. B. Baillière et fils. 3 vols., Fifth edition. (First edition, 2 vols., 1861–1862)*

The collected lectures on clinical medicine presented at the Faculty of Medicine in Paris. The lectures dealing with diseases of the gastrointestinal tract are included in Volume III. On dyspepsia, the author comments: "What has been said about solid foods, holds true also for liquids . . . these should be taken in small amounts and it would be well to insist on fermented beverages, wine and sometimes beer, diluted with water." (pp. 46–47)

1887
Hirtz BOISSONS ALCOOLIQUES: VIN, *in:* NOUVEAU DICTIONNAIRE DE MEDECINE ET DE CHIRURGIE. *Paris: J. B. Baillière et fils.*

In the section on alcohols in this popular medical encyclopedia there appears an article covering briefly the various types of wines used for medical purposes, and including an explanation on the constituents of wine and their therapeutic uses. "In cases of local atony of the stomach . . . a few spoon-fuls of Bordeaux wine . . . combined with a substantial diet and taken immediately after the meal, will work wonders." (p. 613) Furthermore, the author comments: "In nervous vom-iting, iced champagne in small doses is superior to all [other] anti-spasmodics." (p. 613)

1891–1894
Charcot, J. M.; Bouchard, and Brissaud TRAITE DE MEDECINE. *Paris: G. Masson, 6 vols.*

In dilatation of the stomach "red wine is proscribed; one should recommend water to which ¼ white wine or ⅓ beer has been added." (Vol. 3, p. 355) In cancer of the stomach when malnutrition becomes serious, the authors recommend a formula for rectal feeding: 250 gr. bouillon, 120 gr. wine, the yolks of 2 eggs, dry peptone, 5–20 gr. (Vol. 3, p. 390)

1899
Dieulafoy, Georges CLINIQUE MEDICALE DE L'HOTEL-DIEU DE PARIS, 1897–98. *Paris: Masson et Cie., Vol. 2.*

A collection of lectures delivered by the author, in which the various clinical aspects of gastrointestinal diseases are presented and in which case histories and medical treatment are discussed. With regard to peptic ulcer, the author recom-mends—beginning twenty days after surgery—a diet in which both milk and wine are included.

1900
Manquat, A. TRAITE ELEMENTAIRE DE THERAPEUTIQUE, DE MA-TIERE MEDICALE ET DE PHARMACOLOGIE. *Paris: J. B. Baillière et fils, 2 vols., Fourth edition. (First edition, 1892)*

A handbook on therapeusis and therapeutic agents charac-teristic of the period. The first volume deals with therapeutic procedures, and the second with the physiologic effects of vari-ous pharmaceutic agents. "Wines are completely unsuitable to dyspeptics: they [wines] augment gastric acidity and cause heart burn. The light wines with a fairly low content of alco-hol, low content of acids and tannin, are most acceptable, and white wines are preferable to red wines." (Vol. I, p. 926)

1905
Lyon, Gaston TRAITE ELEMENTAIRE DE CLINIQUE THERAPEU-TIQUE. *Paris: Masson & Cie., Sixth edition. (First edition, G. Masson, 1895)*

Written by the retired chairman of the Department of Clinical Medicine, Medical Faculty, Paris, this book discusses the clinical therapeusis of the time. Regarding flatulence, he says: "The permissible liquids are aged wine mixed with water, pure water or a slightly mineral water." (p. 208) In ulcer of the stomach, where rectal feeding becomes necessary, especially after hemorrhage has occurred and before instituting milk treatment, the author recommends the following formula: "250 gm. milk, 2 egg yolks, a pinch of salt, and 1 teaspoonful of red wine. Three such feedings in 24 hours . . ." (p. 271)

1906
Black, John Janvier EATING TO LIVE, WITH SOME ADVICE TO THE GOUTY, THE RHEUMATIC, AND THE DIABETIC; A BOOK FOR EVERYBODY. *Philadelphia: J. B. Lippincott Company.*

"Wine enters the system with no change except being mixed with digestive juices, and absorbs none of the digestive ferments in its own digestion, and hence its usefulness in dyspeptic troubles." (pp. 290–291)

1909
Pascault, L. CONSEILS THEORIQUES ET PRATIQUES SUR L'ALIMENTATION. *Paris: A. Maloine.*

"In gastric motor insufficiency, wine taken in extremely small doses, provides a salutary force in dyspepsia." (p. 78)

Yorke-Davies, N. E. WINE AND HEALTH. HOW TO ENJOY BOTH. *London: Chatto & Windus.*

"In the case of the dyspeptic, . . . weak brandy and water, or pure natural wine, is indicated with the meal." (p. 81)

1921
Arnozan, X., and Jacques Carles PRECIS DE THERAPEUTIQUE. *Paris: G. Doin, Fifth edition. Quoted by F. Dougnac:* LE VIN. *Bordeaux: Editions Delmas, 1935. (p. 255)*

". . . in patients in whom the gastric juice is poor in chlorhydric acid, who are anemic, and have a sluggish digestion, there is nothing more effective than the regular use of a good red Bordeaux wine."

Martinet, Alfred THERAPEUTIQUE CLINIQUE. I. AGENTS THERAPEUTIQUES; II. TECHNIQUES THERAPEUTIQUES; III. TRAITEMENT DES SYMPTOMES; IV. TRAITEMENT DES MALADIES, AVEC LA COLLABORATION DE MM. DESFOSSES, G. LAURENS, LEON MEUNIER,

LOMON, LUTIER, MARTINGAY, MOUGEOT, ET SAINTE-CENE. *Paris: Masson & Cie., 2 vols.*

This textbook is an elaborate exposition of drugs which have a specific effect on a defined organic function, and drugs which act electively in infections. It also discusses dietary and psychic agents; therapeutic techniques; symptomatic therapy; and recommends treatments in the various diseases of organ systems of the human body. The section on diseases of the digestive system is written by Léon Meunier, who recommends in hyposecretion: "Quinine wine . . . or tincture of nux vomica in a glass of Bordeaux wine . . . 10 to 15 minutes before meals." (Vol. 2, p. 1072)

von Friedrich, L., and K. E. Neumann NEUERE ERFAHRUNGEN MIT DEM ALKOHOL-PROBEFRÜHSTÜCK. *Deutsch. Med. Wschr., 47:43.*

A preliminary report on studies in which the alcohol test-meal was used as a test of gastric function. The results indicated the test to be reliable, economical, and simple enough for use by the private practitioner of medicine.

1923

Frehse, K. UEBER DIE WIRKUNG DES ALKOHOLS AUF DIE AZIDITÄT DES MAGENSAFTES UND IHRE DIFFERENTIAL-DIAGNOSTISCHE BEDEUTUNG. *Deutsch. Med. Wschr., 49:11–12.*

A report of an investigation on healthy male subjects, on patients with ulcer, carcinoma, achylia gastrica, nervous dyspepsia and other diseases of the stomach. In all these subjects, the effect of alcohol on the acidity of the gastric juice was observed and recorded. It was found that the acidity was decreased in patients with ulcer and carcinoma; that there was no noticeable response to alcohol in patients with achylia gastrica; but in patients with nervous dyspepsia, gastric acidity was increased after administration of the alcohol.

1931

Doléris, J. A. LE VIN ET LES MEDECINS; LE POUR ET LE CONTRE. *Paris: Vigot frères.*

"Wine is useful in cases where there is an insufficiency of gastric juice." (p. 85)

Kitchin, Kathleen, and D. Harcourt Kitchin, editors A REVIEW OF THE EFFECTS OF ALCOHOL ON MAN. *London: V. Gollancz Ltd.*

"For the rare fermentative conditions of the stomach, and for gastric flatulence, alcohol should be given in the form of brandy, good red wine or dry champagne." (pp. 206–207)

1937
Weissenbach, R. J., and G. Faroy LE VIN ET LE JUS DE RAISIN DANS LA DIETETIQUE ET LE TRAITEMENT DES AFFECTIONS GAS-TRO-INTESTINALES. *IVe Congrès Nat'l. Amis des Vins de France, Alger, pp. 86–158.*

The authors are of the opinion that in hypochlorhydria "wine fulfills the role of a secretory excitant because of its content of alcohol and acids." In hypochlorhydria without gastritis they suggest using a red "vin ordinaire," or old wines low in alcohol and tannin, or slightly sweet wines, 50 cc. to be taken 20–30 minutes before meals, as aperitifs, and the same amount again during the meal, in each case, well diluted with water. (pp. 109–110)

Joffe, P. M., and N. Jolliffe THE GASTRIC ACIDITY IN ALCOHOL ADDICTS WITH OBSERVATIONS ON THE RELATION OF THE B VITA-MINS TO ACHLORHYDRIA. *Am. J. Med. Sci., 193:501–510.*

A study of gastric acidity curves in 105 alcohol addicts (77 males and 28 females) of long standing. The patients were observed under hospital conditions for one week. The results showed achlorhydria in about one-third of all subjects, hypo-chlorhydria in another third, and in one-third adequate secre-tion of free acid was observed. "Achlorhydria was not related to the degree or duration of the alcohol addiction, and did not occur more frequently in subjects having macrocytic anemia or showing the greater degree of liver dysfunction . . . We conclude that: Alcohol *per se* does not cause achlorhydria in the alcohol addict." (p. 509)

1938
Loeper, M., and Ch. Michel FORMULAIRE PRATIQUE DE THERA-PEUTIQUE ET DE PHARMACOLOGIE. ANCIEN FORMULAIRE DE DU-JARDIN-BEAUMETZ. *34th edition. Paris: G. Doin et Cie.*

"White wines, less nourishing than red, but lighter because of their lower content in tannin, are suitable for dyspeptic persons." (p. 577)

1940
Berggren, S. M., and L. Goldberg THE ABSORPTION OF ETHYL ALCOHOL FROM THE GASTROINTESTINAL TRACT AS A DIFFUSION

PROCESS. *Acta Physiol. Scand. 1:246–270.*

A report of an investigation carried out at the Karolinska Institute in Stockholm, in which, by means of direct determinations, the concentration of ethyl alcohol in the stomach during absorption was measured. Three series of experiments were carried out: one on cats, one on normal human subjects, and one on human subjects suffering from achlorhydria and gastritis. It was found that the absorption of ethyl alcohol from the stomach, in all three groups, follows the laws of diffusion—that is, the greater the concentration of alcohol ingested, the more rapidly will the blood alcohol level rise.

McGuigan, Hugh Alister APPLIED PHARMACOLOGY. *St. Louis: The C. V. Mosby Company.*

"In depressive emotional conditions the effects [of small quantities of alcohol on digestion] may be beneficial. The best results are usually secured by wine, perhaps from the psychic effect of the alcoholic content (10–25 per cent) . . . In fatigue also, by diminishing the feeling, [alcohol] acts as an aid to digestion. Taken in moderate quantities in diluted form, before meals, it may be of considerable value in dyspepsia . . . In the form of light wine its use may be beneficial in the atony of the stomach which often follows acute illness, overwork, or in senility." (pp. 260, 429)

1942

Thewlis, Malford W. THE CARE OF THE AGED (GERIATRICS). *St. Louis: The C. V. Mosby Company, Fourth edition.*

"Champagne will often stop vomiting when other measures fail; . . . Now there are other effective methods for correcting these conditions, although champagne is still as effective as the other methods in certain types of vomiting." (p. 144)

1950

Holler, G.; K. Neugebauer, and J. Schmid EIN BEITRAG ZUR MAGENFUNKTION. (SCHLEIMFRAKTIONEN, BLUTHISTAMIN UND AZIDITÄT NACH ALKOHOLBELASTUNG.) *Gastroenterologia (Basel) 76:18–22.*

Fasting healthy human subjects and patients with gastritis and ulcer received 300 cc. of 5% alcohol by stomach tube. The stomach contents were sampled every 15 minutes and the blood every 30 minutes. The mucus fractions, mucoprotein, mucoproteose and mucin in the gastric content, as well as the histamine concentration in the blood, increased in the normal subjects after the administration of alcohol; acidity, on the other hand, lagged somewhat. In patients with gastritis and ulcer, only the mucoproteose and mucin increased; however, the mucoprotein decreased and the blood histamine showed very little variation. The buffer capacity of the mucus fraction in these experiments is discussed.

1951
Motteram, R. A BIOPSY STUDY OF CHRONIC GASTRITIS AND GASTRIC ATROPHY. *J. Path. Bact., 63:389–394.*

A report dealing with histologic studies of tissue biopsy from 150 patients with a variety of dyspeptic symptoms, and some others (43) suffering from pernicious anemia. Among the first group, biopsies were performed on 20 cases of known alcoholism with associated malnutrition. After hospitalization for a period of 2 to 3 weeks, 19 of these subjects showed normal gastric mucosa or only very minor deviations from normal. The gastric mucosa of patients with superficial gastritis due to excess of alcohol returned to normal after withdrawal of the alcohol. In the cases of pernicious amenia, adequate liver therapy failed to alter the pathologic pattern of the mucosa.

CONTRAINDICATIONS

Very little experimental data are available concerning contraindications to the use of wine in disorders of the stomach. Most of the evidence comes from clinical trials and some contradiction exists particularly with regard to the use of wine in dyspepsia. Wines high in acids are best avoided in the presence of hyperchlorhydria.

The prevalent opinion seems to be that wine should be proscribed in cancer, gastritis, and hematemesis. Because of the dearth of experimental evidence it is, of course, prudent to use wine with great caution in any disorder of the stomach and to discontinue its use immediately if any untoward symptom occurs.

1833
Beaumont, William EXPERIMENTS AND OBSERVATIONS ON THE GASTRIC JUICE AND THE PHYSIOLOGY OF DIGESTION. *Plattsburgh: F. P. Allen.*

"The injury which a constant use of wine is known to produce on some stomachs, has been sometimes attributed to the small quantity of tartaric acid which it contains. [But] it is the acidity produced by the acetous fermentation of the saccharine matter contained in the wine, aided, perhaps, by the alcohol which is in a state of combination with it [which is responsible for the injury to the stomach]. (p. 50)

1873

Becquerel, A. TRAITE ELEMENTAIRE D'HYGIENE PRIVEE ET PUBLIQUE. *Paris: P. Asselin, Fifth edition.*

The author states, relative to the stomach, that "Acid wines of cold climates are bad for the stomach, producing gastric disturbances, dyspepsia, and often diarrhea." (p. 684)

1876

Richardson, (Sir) Benjamin W. ON ALCOHOL. A COURSE OF SIX CANTOR LECTURES DELIVERED BEFORE THE SOCIETY OF ARTS. *New York: The National Temperance Society and Publication House.*

"Of all the systems of organs, those that suffer most [from alcohol] are the digestive and the nervous systems. The stomach, unable to produce in proper quantity the natural digestive fluid, is in constant anxiety and irritation. It is oppressed with the sense of nausea; it is oppressed with a sense of distention; it is oppressed with a loathing for food and it is teased with a craving for more drink. Thus there is engendered a permanent disorder which for politeness' sake is called dyspepsia, and for which different remedies are often sought but never found. (pp. 154–155)

1905

Lyon, Gaston TRAITE ELEMENTAIRE DE CLINIQUE THERAPEUTIQUE. *Paris: Masson & Cie., Sixth edition.*

On dyspepsia, the author comments: "In general, dyspeptics do not take wine very well, it increases the stomach acidity; wine is contraindicated in hyperchlorhydria and where acetic fermentation is present. [When tolerated] white wine is preferable to red . . . sparkling wines should always be prohibited." (p. 117)

1909

Yorke-Davies, N. E. WINE AND HEALTH. HOW TO ENJOY BOTH. *London: Chatto & Windus.*

On dyspepsia, the author comments: "Sweet wines of all descriptions should be avoided." (p. 81)

1921

Arnozan, X., and Jacques Carles PRECIS DE THERAPEUTIQUE.

Paris: G. Doin, Fifth edition. Quoted by F. Dougnac: LE VIN.
Bordeaux: Editions Delmas, 1935. (p. 255)

"As far as diseases of the stomach are concerned . . . it is best to avoid a wine very high in acids and tannin."

1931
Doleris, J. A. LE VIN ET LES MEDECINS; LE POUR ER LE CONTRE. *Paris: Vigot frères.*

"Wine is contraindicated in stomach ulcers or tumors and in dyspepsia linked with hyperchlorhydria. (p. 80)

1937
Weissenbach, R. J., and G. Faroy LE VIN ET LE JUS DE RAISIN DANS LA DIETETIQUE ET LE TRAITEMENT DES AFFECTIONS GASTRO-INTESTINALES. *IVe Congrès Nat'l. Méd. Amis des Vins de France, Alger, pp. 86–158.*

"In cases of gastritis, carcinoma of the stomach, and pernicious anemia, wine should be strictly forbidden . . . [In hyperchlorhydria] highly acidic wines, sweet wines, and wines high in alcohol must be proscribed." (pp. 109, 111)

1943
Stryjenski, L. KREBS UND ALKOHOLISMUS. *Schweiz. Med. Wschr., 73:1526–1530.*

A report based on findings at autopsy, covering some 50 years experience and about 5800 autopsies. The conclusion drawn is that the use of alcohol and tobacco may be etiologically significant in the prevalence of cancer of the stomach and esophagus among the male population.

1956
Williams, A. W. EFFECTS OF ALCOHOL ON THE GASTRIC MUCOSA. *Brit. Med. J., 1:256–259.*

Histological studies of stomach tissues obtained from 25 alcoholic subjects, as follows: biopsy 16, postgastrectomy 25, and necropsy 6, and a report of experimental studies on the effects of alcohol on the stomachs of guinea pigs. The histological studies showed the stomach mucosa to be frequently normal and indicated that the relationship of alcoholism to chronic gastritis is uncertain. In the animal experiments, alcohol in concentrations equal to that of gin or whiskey caused severe hemorrhagic and ulcerative lesions.

4 The Effects of Wine and its Constituents on the Functions and Disorders of the Intestines

EFFECTS ON NORMAL FUNCTIONS

Anatomically, the intestine is divided into two sections: the small and the large intestine. The small intestine comprises the duodenum, jejunum and the ileum; the large intestine includes the cecum, colon, rectum and the anal canal.

The small intestine is a long tubular tract, disposed in coils which occupy an important share of the abdominal cavity. It is attached to the posterior wall of the cavity by a membraneous tissue which supplies it with blood. Two layers of muscle, one circular and one longitudinal, provide the peristaltic motion essential to propelling the chyme along the tube. The peristaltic movement is continuous but varies in intensity, depending upon the amount of chyme within the intestine. The interior wall is lined by a villi-containing membrane, each villus consisting of a stem composed of lymph channels and several capillaries. A single layer of mucus-secreting cells separates the chyme from the lymph channels and capillaries. Functionally, the small intestine is divided into three sections: the duodenum, the jejunum and the ileum.

The duodenum is that part of the small intestine where important digestive processes take place. It is the C-shaped por-

tion which curves from the pyloric end of the stomach downward and to the right, and then doubles back to the left side.
When the partially digested food from the stomach—the chyme—
enters the duodenum through the pylorus, the mucus-secreting
cells produce and pour forth secretin—an enzyme which activates the pancreas. The bile from the liver and gall bladder and
the enzymes collected from the pancreas are secreted into the
downward limb of the duodenum there to assist in the further
breakdown of the chyme. Proteins are converted into amino
acids, fats into fatty acids and glycerol, and carbohydrates into
simple sugars.

The jejunum and the ileum are the segments where the major part of absorption occurs. The simple substances of the now
completely broken down chyme are absorbed through the semi-
permeable villous membrane through physico-chemical processes,
and transferred to the blood and lymph channels. Veins drain-
ing the intestine carry these materials into the portal vein and
thus to the liver.

The cecum, the vestibule of the large intestine, drains the
ileum. It stretches upward from the lower right corner of the
abdomen and after a right-angle turn becomes the transverse
colon, crossing the abdomen below the liver, and then bends
downward and to the left to become the rectum and finally the
anal canal.

The large intestine, though short in length when compared
to the small intestine, is about twice the diameter of the latter.
Its muscular wall resembles that of the small intestine but the
mucosal wall is relatively simpler since it does not contain an
overt villous structure and no enzyme-secreting cells. However,
a copious amount of mucus is secreted in this segment of the
bowel. No digestion of food and almost no absorption—except
of water—occurs in the large intestine.

In the cecum and colon numerous bacteria reside. They are
active in the production of vitamin K—a substance essential to
the blood coagulation equilibrium. In addition, several components of the vitamin B complex are produced, while vitamin C
is destroyed by these bacterial inhabitants of the large bowel.
Here also, most of the water, admixed to the chyme, is removed.
The residue which reaches the rectum as fecal matter, is composed of bacteria, some chemical substances, and disintegrat-
ing leukocytes and lining tissues. In the rectum, mucus is produced which facilitates the passage of fecal material through the
anal canal and its sphincters.

Most of the research on the effects of wine and its constituents on the intestine concerns problems of motility, absorption, and secretion. In addition, the role of wine as a bactericidal agent has received much attention. Kuno (1914) found that very small concentrations of methyl and ethyl alcohol stimulate intestinal peristalsis; Wallace and Jackson (1902) found that a 25% solution of alcohol injected into the intestine greatly stimulates gastric secretion. It was Dragstedt and coworkers (1940) who ascribed the stimulating effect to the histamine-like action of alcohol. Hanzlik and Collins (1913) found that a 10% solution of alcohol is absorbed more efficiently than either a 5, 50 or a 95% solution. Edkins (1926) is of the opinion that alcohol is more rapidly absorbed in the presence of CO_2.

The first experimental study on the bactericidal effect of wine was done by Professor Pick (1892) of Vienna, and it was followed by many similar investigations in the more important research centers of the Western world. It was established that wine had a definite bactericidal action and that this was not due to its content of alcohol. Masquelier and coworker (1953) ascribed the bactericidal effect of wine to its content of anthocyanins and related pigments. Powers and his group (1960) obtained similar results and ascribed the bactericidal effect of wine to its content of colorless leucobase.

1892
Pick, A. UEBER DEN EINFLUSS DES WEINES AUF DIE ENTWICKE-LUNG DES TYPHUS- UND CHOLERA-BACILLEN. *Zentralbl. f. Bakt. u. Parasitenk., 12:293–294.*

Cultures of typhus and cholera bacilli were prepared and the bactericidal activity of the following solutions tested: 10 g. water + 10 g. white wine; 20 g. white wine; 10 g. red wine + 10 g. water; 20 g. red wine; and 20 g. sterile water as the control solution. The author noted that the bacterial cultures continued to survive for prolonged periods of time in the control solution, whereas in the wine and in the wine and water mixtures the bacterial growth began to decelerate within 2 hours and all the bacilli were dead within 24 hours. Professor Pick recommended, as a preventive and therapeutic measure, the addition of wine to drinking water well ahead of its consumption, particularly in times of epidemics.

1902
Wallace, G. B., and H. C. Jackson IS THE ACTION OF ALCOHOL

ON GASTRIC SECRETION SPECIFIC? *Amer. J. Physiol. (Proceedings), 8:XVII–XVIII.*

The authors give a brief report of experiments on dogs designed to elucidate the mechanisms by which alcohol introduced into the intestine affects the flow of gastric juice. "40 cc. of 25 per cent alcohol, injected into the intestine, produced a gastric flow five times as great in amount as when water alone was injected . . . 0.3 cc. of oil of peppermint, . . . produced an effect practically identical with that of alcohol . . . The conclusions are (1) that alcohol introduced into the intestine stimulates the gastric secretions not through its absorption and subsequent action on the gastric mucosa, but by a purely reflex action; (2) that this action is not limited to alcohol, but is possessed by other irritant substances, such as oil of peppermint." (p. XVIII)

1903
Chittenden, R. H. THE INFLUENCE OF ALCOHOL AND ALCOHOLIC BEVERAGES ON DIGESTION AND SECRETION. IN: PHYSIOLOGICAL ASPECTS OF THE LIQUOR PROBLEM. *John S. Billings, editor. New York: Houghton, Mifflin and Company, Vol. 1, pp. 137–305.*

In this article is recorded one of the earliest experiments on the effects of alcoholic beverages on the digestive system, in vitro, and on human subjects. The results showed that alcoholic beverages in general stimulate the secretion of a concentrated gastric juice, both directly and indirectly, through the influence of the alcohol absorbed directly from the intestines. Wine showed an inhibitory effect on proteolysis which was neutralized, however, by the increase in gastric flow. Among his conclusions, the author agrees with Sir William Roberts that "a glass or two of claret, hock or sherry with dinner or luncheon would evidently not produce any appreciable retardation of peptic action, but would . . . act as pure stimulants." (pp. 150–151)

1905
Wetmore, C. A. THE RATIONAL USE OF WINES IN HEALTH AND DISEASE. *Pacific Med. Surg. J., 48:593–598.*

Following his return from Europe, the author, a physician who became converted to the medicinal uses of wine while on his trip, advised for therapeutic purposes the substitution of a light, slightly acid wine instead of the stronger liquors. The author recommended, particularly in those regions where dysentery prevails, a claret punch composed of claret and water with added lemon juice, to be taken at least once a day.

1907

Sabrazès, J., and A. Marcandier ACTION DU VIN SUR LE BACILLE D'EBERTH. *Ann. Inst. Pasteur, 21:312–320.*

The bactericidal effect of various wines on Eberthella was tested. Both red and white wines, French and Algerian, were used in this experiment. It was noted that white wine was effective within 6 hours and red within 12 hours. The superiority of white wine as a bactericidal agent was not explained. The authors suggest that white or red wine be added to the water 6 to 12 hours before drinking it.

1913

Hanzlik, P. J., and R. J. Collins QUANTITATIVE STUDIES ON THE GASTROINTESTINAL ABSORPTION OF DRUGS. III. THE ABSORPTION OF ALCOHOL. *J. Pharmacol. Exp. Ther., 5:185–213.*

A report of studies on cats and dogs wherein the gastrointestinal absorption of alcohol was measured and compared. It was found that the "absorption of alcohol is scarcely influenced by the concentration of the alcohol, although a 10 per cent solution is absorbed somewhat better than 5, 50 and 95 per cent solutions." However, when a simultaneous injection of alcohol is delivered intravenously, the absorption from the intestine is inhibited "due to a slowing of the circulation in the intestine." (p. 213)

1914

Kuno, Y. UEBER DIE WIRKUNG DER EINWERTIGEN ALKOHOLE AUF DEN ÜBERLEBENDEN KANINCHENDARM. *Arch. Exp. Path. Pharm., 77:206–217.*

The author reports a study of the effects of methyl, ethyl, propyl, butyl, and amyl alcohols on the isolated intestine of rabbits. The results indicate that in the smallest concentrations possible, methyl and ethyl alcohol stimulate intestinal motility, while propyl, butyl and amyl alcohol, after an initial period of stimulation, had a paralyzing effect.

1920

Coronado, C. E. A. FALSIFICATIONS DU VIN ET L'ALCOOLISME. *Paris: Thesis #336.*

A quaint report, usual for such theses, records "a young

Parisian woman whose gastric digestion had been subject to difficulties for many years (cramps, continual heart burn, etc.), while her intestinal digestion was excellent, was cured in less than 2 months by the regular and moderate use of a wine of Médoc." (p. 271)

1923
Ivy, A. C., and G. B. McIlvain THE EXCITATION OF GASTRIC SECRETION BY APPLICATION OF SUBSTANCES TO THE DUODENAL AND JEJUNAL MUCOSA. *Amer. J. Physiol., 67:124–140.*

A report of experiments in which a variety of substances were applied directly to the duodenal and jejunal mucosa of dogs which had been prepared with a Pavlov or Heidenhain pouch. The resulting gastric secretion was collected, measured and analyzed. Among the substances used were hydrochloric acid, 10% ethyl alcohol, glucose and histamine. The results indicated that the 10% solution of ethyl alcohol was one of the most active and most constant excitants of gastric secretion.

1926
Edkins, N., and M. M. Murray THE EFFECT OF CO_2 ON THE ABSORPTION OF ALCOHOL AND THE INFLUENCE OF ALCOHOL ON THE DIFFUSION OF CO_2 IN THE SMALL INTESTINE. *J. Physiol., 62:13–16.*

In serial experiments decerebrated cats received unbuffered Ringer solution (control), Ringer $+$ 8% alcohol, and Ringer $+$ 8% alcohol $+$ about 44% CO_2, and their absorption was observed and measured. "With regard to the absorption of alcohol in the presence of CO_2, there seems to be a tendency for more alcohol to be absorbed [from the intestine] in the presence of CO_2, though the effect is not nearly so marked as in the stomach." (p. 15)

1927
Rolleston, J. D. ALCOHOLISM IN CLASSICAL ANTIQUITY. *Brit. J. Inebriety, 24:101–120.*

A review of the drinking mores of the ancients, with quotes from Athenaeus, Pliny, and Galen. The review deals primarily with alcoholism, preventive measures and cures. A passing remark is concerned with the physiologic effects of alcoholic beverages, i.e., "certain wines were looked on with disfavour, such as 'abates' . . . which had no effect beyond that of relaxing the bowels." (p. 103)

1930
Cori, C. F.; E. L. Villiaume, and G. T. Cori STUDIES ON INTES-
TINAL ABSORPTION. II. THE ABSORPTION OF ETHYL ALCOHOL. *J.
Biol. Chem., 87:19–25.*

The authors report their experimental studies from the Institute for the Study of Malignant Disease at Buffalo, New
York. Investigation on rats were carried out to determine the
capacity of the intestinal tract regarding the absorption of
alcohol. It was found that "the rate of absorption of alcohol
depends on and is roughly parallel to the amount fed [and
that] up to a 20% solution the concentration has little influence on the rate of absorption. A 40% solution of alcohol is
absorbed more slowly than a 20% solution due to slow evacuation of the stomach . . . The rate of emptying of the stomach
is the determining factor for the rate of absorption of alcohol
[from the intestine]." (p. 24)

1933
Kling, A., and D. Florentin ROLE QUE PEUVENT JOUER LES
BOISSONS ACIDS ET ALCOOLIQUES DANS LA PROPHYLAXIE DE LA
FIÈVRE TYPHOIDE. *Bull. Acad. Med., 110:310–322.*

A report of experiments carried out at the Municipal Laboratory of Paris. The efficacy of various acid and alcoholic
beverages to act as bactericides was tested. The beverages included orange and lemon juice with and without alcohol,
commercial lemonades, wines, yogurts, and various aperitifs.
Among the beverages capable of rendering polluted water
safe for drinking, wine was the most efficient, particularly
vins ordinaires of average brisk acidity.

1937
Remlinger, P., and J. Bailly ACTION DU VIN SUR LES BACILLES
DE LA DYSENTERIE. *Rev. Hyg., 59:365–368.*

The bactericidal effect of a variety of wines on dysentery
bacilli was studied. It was noted that the efficacy of wine
varied slightly from one variety to another, but that all of the
white wines were more active than the red wines. The authors
suggest that possibly the tannins are responsible for the bactericidal effect of wine, despite the fact that red wines are
richer in tannin than white wines.

1940
Dybing, O., and E. W. Rasmussen DIE RESORPTION DES ÄTHYL-
ALKOHOLS AUS DEM MAGEN UND DARM DER RATTE. *Biochem. Z.,
306:337–342.*

A report of experimental studies from the Institute of Pharmacy of the University of Oslo. Male white rats received 5, 10, 20 and 40% solutions of alcohol (intraperitoneally and perorally) after a 36-hour period of starvation during which time they had access to fluids. It was found that resorption of the lower concentrations of alcohol occurred from the stomach, but that blood levels corresponding to the higher concentrations of alcohol were found after intestinal resorption.

Dragstedt, C. A.; J. S. Gray; A. H. Lawton, and M. Ramirez deArellano DOES ALCOHOL STIMULATE GASTRIC SECRETION BY LIBERATING HISTAMINE? *Proc. Soc. Exp. Biol. Med., 43:26–28.*

A report of experimental studies to determine whether alcohol could liberate histamine from tissues, thus giving a valid basis to the concept that alcohol acts through a "histaminegic" mechanism. Isolated lungs of guinea pigs were used in these studies. Five cc. of 5, 7, and 15% alcohol solutions were injected into the perfusion system, or the control perfusion fluid was replaced by perfusion fluids containing 2, 3, 4, or 6% alcohol. The histamine-like activity of the perfusate was tested on guinea pig intestine. After addition of the alcohol by either method, an increase in the histamine-like activity of the perfusate occurred. It was felt that this activity was due to histamine because it was destroyed by boiling the perfusate while alkaline but not when acid; by incubation with histaminase. "The stimulating action of the perfusate upon the guinea pig intestine is not prevented by atropine, but is prevented by arginin. While the identification of the active substance in the perfusates as histamine is not absolute, it is certainly very strong." (p. 27)

1941

Adler, H. F.; J. M. Beazell; A. J. Atkinson, and A. C. Ivy THE MOTOR RESPONSE OF THE COLON TO ALCOHOL. *Quart. J. Stud. Alc., 1:638–644.*

Some experiments carried out at the Department of Physiology and Pharmacology, Northwestern University Medical School (Chicago) are reported. The effect of alcohol on the motility of the colon was determined in 4 dogs and 2 adult males who had just undergone colostomy. From the results obtained, the authors conclude that alcohol in the quantities used (200–250 cc. of 20% alcohol) tends to alter the type of colonic motility of man without greatly influencing the amount of motility.

Ettinger, G. H.; A. B. Brown, and A. H. Megill POTENTIATION OF ACETYLCHOLINE BY ALCOHOL AND ETHER. *J. Pharmacol. Exp. Ther., 73:119–126.*

A report of experimental studies, from the Department of Physiology, Queen's University (Ontario), in which an attempt is made "to relate the degree to which the effect of acetylcholine on the frog's rectus abdominis may be magnified, if the acetylcholine is dissolved in varying strengths of ethyl alcohol or diethyl ether, before being added to the bath containing the rectus." (p. 119) The results of the experiments indicated that "solutions of acetylcholine in ethyl alcohol and diethyl ether cause greater contraction of the frog rectus than do aqueous solutions . . ." Similar experiments were carried out on rabbit's intestine and it was found that "solutions of acetylcholine in alcohol or ether cause less stimulation of the rabbit's intestine than do aqueous solutions." (p. 125)

1952

Koskowski, W., and M. Mahfouz THE EFFECTS OF ALCOHOL ON THE SECRETION OF INTESTINAL JUICE AND THE ACTIVITY OF INVERTASE. *Gastroenterology, 21:286–288.*

A report of experiments carried out in Egypt at Farouk I University in which the authors attempted to examine the effect of alcohol on intestinal secretion and its invertase activity, and to see if these effects could be altered by the administration of a potent antihistamine. The experiments were carried out on dogs. The alcohol was administered by stomach tube (300 cc. of 7% solution) and intravenously (10 cc. of 30% solution). It was found that the action of ethyl alcohol in stimulating secretion was similar to that of histamine and that a potent antihistaminic drug ("Anthisan") had an antagonistic effect.

1953

Beck, L. C. DUODENAL ULCER IN HAWAII. *Proc. Straub Clin., 19:161–166. (Abstract in: Quart. J. Stud. Alc., 15:517, 1954).*

"The racial distribution of 91 patients with duodenal ulcer admitted to the Straub Clinic in Honolulu paralleled that in the general population . . . among the Caucasians 20 (50%) were users of alcohol to the extent of 4 oz. of liquor per week or more; among the Japanese only 2 (12%) used alcohol. There seems to be no relationship between race or use of alcohol and incidence of duodenal ulcer. The use of caffeine, tobacco and alcohol may be the first expression of anxiety and maladjustment but in themselves these substances are not direct causes of ulcer."

Gardner, J. ON THE ANTIBACTERIAL PROPERTIES OF WINE. PRE-SENTED BEFORE THE AMERICAN PHARMACEUTICAL ASSOCIATION, SALT LAKE CITY, AUGUST 19. *Quoted by* SALVATORE PABLO LU-CIA: A HISTORY OF WINE AS THERAPY. *Philadelphia: J. B. Lippincott Company, 1963. (p. 179)*

A series of experiments on the bactericidal effects of wine on three species of bacteria: Staphylococcus aureus; Escherichia coli; and Bacillus megatherium. Wine proved an effective bactericidal agent for these microorganisms. This property of wine was due neither to its content of alcohol, aldehydes, tannins, nor to its content of acids. In further experiments with dealcoholized wine, the author succeeded in isolating a compound, soluble in alcohol and in water, which completely inhibited the growth of Staphylococcus aureus and Bacillus megatherium. The author described the compound as a "wine antibiotic," but was unable to identify it chemically.

Masquelier, J., and H. Jensen RECHERCHES SUR L'ACTION BAC-TERICIDE DES VINS ROUGES. *Bull. Soc. Pharm. Bordeaux, 91: 24–29; 105–109.*

A series of studies on the bactericidal properties of red wines in an attempt to identify the active ingredient in the wine. Their results indicated that the anthocyanins and related pigments of wine are responsible for its bactericidal effect and that these substances become active only after fermentation of the grape occurs.

1960
Pratt, D. E.; J. J. Powers, and D. Somaatmadja ANTHOCYANINS. I. THE INFLUENCE OF STRAWBERRY AND GRAPE ANTHOCYANINS ON THE GROWTH OF CERTAIN BACTERIA. *Food Res., 25:26–32.*
> *and*

Powers, J. J.; D. Somaatmadja; D. E. Pratt, and M. K. Hamdy ANTHOCYANINS. II. THE ACTION OF ANTHOCYANIN PIGMENTS AND RELATED COMPOUNDS ON THE GROWTH OF CERTAIN MICROOR-GANISMS. *Food Technol., XIV:626–632.*

Anthocyanin fractions extracted from Pinot Noir wine, from bottled Concord grape juice and from frozen strawberries, were tested on Escherichia coli, Staphylococcus aureus, and Lactobacillus casei. The results showed that some of the fractions, primarily the colorless leucobases from wine, inhibited the growth of the test organisms; while other fractions, which might have retained traces of sugar, appeared to stimulate growth of microorganisms.

1964
Powers, J. J. ACTION OF ANTHOCYANIN AND RELATED COMPOUNDS ON BACTERIAL CELLS. *Publication No. 368, College Experiment Station, College of Agriculture, University of Georgia, Athens, Georgia. (also) 4th International Symposium on Food Microbiology, SIK, Göteborg, Sweden, pp. 59–75.*

The series of studies described indicate that anthocyanin and related compounds are diverse in their action toward bacteria. Of more than 20 anthocyanins investigated, no compound was devoid of activity toward the ten bacteria used as test organisms.

1965
Somaatmadja, D.; J. J. Powers, and R. Wheeler ACTION OF LEUCOANTHOCYANINS OF CABERNET GRAPES ON REPRODUCTION AND RESPIRATION OF CERTAIN BACTERIA. *Amer. J. Enol. Vitic., 16:54–61.*

EFFECTS ON ABNORMAL FUNCTIONS
Intestinal disorders occur frequently and can be due to infections, obstructions, inflammations, or to a functional disturbance in the gastrointestinal tract. Specific research on the effects of wine in these disorders is sparse, and most of the data available concern diarrhea. The use of wine as a therapeutic agent in diarrhea has been known to physicians since antiquity. Hippocrates was perhaps the first to record that a wine high in tannin is effective in alleviating diarrhea, and recent observations have confirmed this hypothesis. Pinel, Stockton, Black, and others, all commented on the beneficial results obtained from the use of a "generous red wine" in the treatment of severe diarrhea.

As stated in the previous section, the antibacterial activity of wine has been firmly established. From this point of view, it is prudent to recommend the use of wine in most intestinal infections. Sollier (1934) recommends wine with meals or wine mixed with water as the liquid of choice in order to combat the activity of the colon bacilli in the intestinal tract.

One important area of research has been the effect of wine in the malabsorption syndrome. The study of Althausen (1960) indicates that certain white wines double the absorption of fat and are thus valuable aids in the treatment of this condition.

1810

Pinel, P. NOSOGRAPHIE PHILOSOPHIQUE; OU, LA METHODE DE L'ANALYSE APPLIQUEE A LA MEDECINE. *Paris: J. A. Brosson, 3 vols., Fourth edition. (First edition, Paris: Maradan, 2 vols., "an VI," [1798]).*

Written by a great humanist held responsible for the more rational treatment of the insane, these volumes constitute an extensive philosophic nosography. In discussing the treatment of dysentery, the author recommends:

> "1. milk and farinaceous substances . . .
>
> 2. an occasional laxative . . .
>
> 3. some astringents and tonics . . .
>
> 4. moderate exercise, fresh air, a diet predominant in dairy products and moderate use of generous wines." (Vol. 2, p. 254)

1817

Loebenstein-Loebel, Ed. TRAITE SUR L'USAGE ET LES EFFETS DES VINS . . . *Strasbourg: F. G. Levrault.*

With regard to diseases of the intestine, the author states: "In intestinal colic with extreme weakness, one should use white wine." (p. 79)

1824

Kitchiner, William THE ART OF INVIGORATING AND PROLONGING LIFE . . . *London: Hurst, Robinson, and Co., Fifth edition.*

In diarrhea, the diet should include "toast and water with about one-fourth part of Wine, and a little Sugar and grated Nutmeg or Ginger in it." (pp. 268–269)

1859

Ollier, L. F. A. ESSAI D'OENOLOGIE MEDICALE. *Strasbourg: Thesis #466.*

For chronic and atonic diarrhea, wine should be used therapeutically "in the form of anemas—the wine to be used to be lightly astringent, old Bordeaux being the best." (p. 38)

1877

Anstie, Francis E. ON THE USES OF WINES IN HEALTH AND DISEASE. *London: Macmillan and Co.*

For diarrhea, the author recommends: "Somewhat more frequently is this kind of wine [effervescent] useful in the catarrhal diarrhea . . . of summer and autumn . . . But if the diarrhea obstinately continues for several days . . . then the greatest benefit will often result from putting him [the patient] upon a ration of ten or twelve ounces of champagne daily, discontinuing all medicines." (pp. 47–48)

Burdel, Edouard LE VIN DANS LA SOLOGNE CONSIDERE COMME PROPHYLACTIQUE PUISSANT DES FIÈVRES TELLURIQUES, LETTRES MEDICALES. *Paris: G. Masson.*
 "Hot wine and spirits are best for the control of chills, vomiting, dysentery, and choleric cramps." (p. 16)

1887
Gustafson, Axel THE FOUNDATION OF DEATH. A STUDY OF THE DRINK QUESTION. *New York: Funk & Wagnalls, Third edition.*
 "Considered in its true character, as a narcotic, the power of alcohol to deaden pain is unquestionable. In colic, . . . a draught of hot water with alcohol no doubt relieves the pain, but it accomplishes this by deadening the nerves. It provokes a more copious flow of the gastric juice, with the immediate effect of facilitating the interrupted digestion." (p. 201)

1889
Herpin, J. C. LA VIGNE ET LE RAISIN. HISTOIRE BOTANIQUE ET CHIMIQUE. EFFETS PHYSIOLOGIQUES ET THERAPEUTIQUES. *Paris: J. B. Baillière et fils.*
 "While taking the grape cure, if constipated, drink a little wine." (p. 279)

1891–1894
Charcot, J. M.; Bouchard, and Brissaud TRAITE DE MEDECINE. *Paris: G. Masson, 6 vols.*
 Discussing intestinal hemorrhage, the authors recommend: "Where collapse is present, the patient should be given wines high in alcohol and subcutaneous injections of ether." (Volume 3, p. 561)

1906
Black, John Janvier EATING TO LIVE . . . *Philadelphia: J. B. Lippincott Company.*
 "Port wine . . . is an astringent wine and is used in diarrheas when wine is indicated." (p. 298)

1907
Cayla, F. REGIMES PATHOLOGIQUES ET REGIME PARFAIT. *Paris: Vigot frères.*

"In diseases of the digestive system such as gastritis, enteritis, enterocolitis, we suggest—with the evening meal—red Bordeaux wine in winter and white in summer, diluted with ½ to ¾ water." (p. 44)

1909
Yorke-Davies, N. E. WINE AND HEALTH. HOW TO ENJOY BOTH. *London: Chatto & Windus.*

For constipation, the author recommends: "All those wines that contain tannin should be studiously avoided . . . The victim of constipation would do best by drinking light white wines, such as Chablis, Sauternes, Hocks, Moselles, Barsac, Barzovah (a dry Cyprus sherry), and dry cider." (p. 89)

1921
Stockton, C. G. EFFECT OF ALCOHOL IN THERAPY OF INTERNAL DISEASES. *Med. Rec., 100:277–279.*

"In chronic diarrhea, where there is hyperperistalsis, . . . a properly selected alcoholic preparation not merely gives comfort to the patient, but at times is positively a live-saving agent for which there is no satisfactory substitute." (p. 278)

1931
Kitchin, Kathleen, and D. Harcourt Kitchin, editors A REVIEW OF THE EFFECTS OF ALCOHOL ON MAN. *London: V. Gollancz Ltd.*

"For the rare fermentative conditions of the stomach, and for gastric flatulence, alcohol should be given in the form of brandy, good red wine, or dry champagne." (pp. 206–207)

1934
Sollier, N. ROLE DU VIN DANS LA PROPHYLAXIE DES COLIBACILLOSES. *IIe Congrès Nat'l. Méd. Amis des Vins de France, Beziers, pp. 179–183.*

Experiments are described in which the bactericidal activity of wine was studied. Two series of experiments were carried out. In the first, an emulsion of water and colon bacilli recently isolated from urine samples was mixed in such a way that each drop of emulsion contained about 100 bacilli. This emulsion was then distributed into 3 test tubes: the first one containing 1 drop of emulsion, plus 1 cc. of water (control); the second containing 1 cc. of water, plus 1 cc. of wine, plus 1 drop of emulsion; and the third containing 1 cc. of wine, plus 1 drop of emulsion. These were then cultured, after 15- and

30-minute contact, in Petri dishes. In the second series polluted water (containing about 500,000 colon bacilli per liter) was mixed with white and red wine in various proportions and cultured as above after 30-minute contact. It was found that wine had a marked antibacterial power, white wine more so than red. In concluding, the author recommends mixing water with wine before drinking, or drinking pure wine with meals, in order to combat the activity of the colon bacilli in the intestinal tract.

1935
Puntoni, V. CONTRIBUTION AU TRAITEMENT PAR LE VIN. *Ier Congrès Comité Méd. Int. pour la Propaganda du Vin, Lausanne.*
One particular case of summer diarrhea is described which remained unchanged after treatment with opiates, bismuth, and tannic acid for one week; and yet the cure was accomplished in a few hours after ingestion of a generous quantity of dry wine excessively rich in tannin. (p. 98)

1937
Weissenbach, R. J., and G. Faroy LE VIN ET LE JUS DE RAISIN DANS LA DIETETIQUE ET LE TRAITEMENT DES AFFECTIONS GASTROINTESTINALES. *IVe Congrès Nat'l. Méd. Amis des Vins de France, Alger, pp. 86–158.*
"Wine has a favorable effect on intestinal digestion . . . It possesses antiseptic properties and is therefore useful in intestinal diseases." (pp. 124–125)

1938
Puntoni, V. LE VIN, VINISME ET ALCOOLISME. *2me Congrès. Int. Méd. pour l'Etude Scient. du Raisin et du Vin, Lisbonne, pp. 52–79.*
"The use of wine in infectious diseases of the gastrointestinal system . . . favors gastrointestinal leukopedesis and activates leukocyte function. In such cases, wine taken in moderate doses can be considered as a general activator of phagocytes." (p. 61)

1940
Beckers, R. THE NUTRITIVE VALUE OF WINE. *Wines & Vines, 21:14, 26.*
"The use of wine as a nutrient may be considered as . . . a regulator of the digestive functions . . . Wine is an antiseptic. The most virulent bacteria, such as the bacillus of typhoid

fever, of dysentery, or of cholera, succumb to its action. They are destroyed within periods varying from five minutes and two hours . . . Therefore it is prudent always, in drinking water the purity of which is doubtful, to dilute water with wine." (p. 14)

1960
Althausen, T. L.; K. Uyeyama, and M. R. Loran EFFECTS OF ALCOHOL ON ABSORPTION OF VITAMIN A IN NORMAL AND GASTRECTOMIZED SUBJECTS. *Gastroenterology, 38:942–945.*

Twenty-four hospital patients, recovering from partial gastrectomy and suffering from malabsorption syndrome, received a regular dose of white wine with their postoperative diet. Absorption of fat was measured by the amount of absorption of Vitamin A. The authors state that the rate of absorption increased from 35 to 431 per cent, averaging 125 per cent.

1965
Goodman, Louis S., and Alfred Gilman, editors THE PHARMACOLOGICAL BASIS OF THERAPEUTICS. *New York: The Macmillan Company, Third edition.*

"In cases of flatulence and colic, alcohol may give relief." (p. 152)

CONTRAINDICATIONS

In certain disorders of the intestine all alcoholic beverages are best proscribed, although there is little direct evidence for the objection. The most obvious condition in which wine is inadvisable is peptic ulcer. It should be kept in mind, however, that the tranquilizing effect of wine can be an effective prophylactic when the ulcer is tension-related. Because of the astringent quality of tannin, it is best that wines high in this substance be prohibited to persons suffering from chronic constipation.

1900
Manquat, A. TRAITE ELEMENTAIRE DE THERAPEUTIQUE, DE MATIERE MEDICALE ET DE PHARMACOLOGIE. *Paris: J. B. Baillière et fils, 2 vols., Fourth edition.*

Discussing disorders of the intestine, the author states: "Wine is absorbed almost in its entirety and may be prescribed as a stimulant; however, care must be exercised since irritation of the intestine may occur . . . One must avoid enemas of pure wine, particularly if the wine is high in tannin." (Vol. I, p. 713)

1909
Yorke-Davies, N. E. WINE AND HEALTH. HOW TO ENJOY BOTH. *London: Chatto & Windus.*

The author recommends for persons who suffer from persistent constipation, a ration of whiskey well diluted with water. "All those wines that contain tannin should be studiously avoided." The patient would do best to drink "light white wines, such as Chablis, Sauternes, Hocks . . ." (p. 89)

1928
Milanesi, E. AZIONE DELL'ALCOOL ETILICO SULL'INTESTINO DI MAMMIFERO. *Arch. Sci. Biol., 2:55–62.*

The author is of the opinion that alcohol has no direct effect on the sympathetic nervous system inasmuch as the effect of adrenalin is not altered; however, excessive amounts of alcohol may have an effect on the muscular layer of the intestine because, in the presence of alcohol, barium chloride acts only incompletely. Nothing precludes the possibility that excessive amounts of alcohol might depress the intestine not only through the muscular layer but also through its intrinsic plexus of nerves.

5 The Effects of Wine and its Constituents on the Functions and Disorders of the Liver and Gallbladder

EFFECTS ON NORMAL FUNCTIONS

The liver, the "most impressive organ in the body," has earned this name not only because of its size—which is four times that of the heart—but primarily because it is the hub from which emanate a variety of functions necessary to maintain the body in equilibrium.

The liver is located in the upper right quadrant of the abdominal cavity and its fine end points toward the stomach. It contains an extensive network of small masses of cells called lobules and it is amply supplied with blood vessels, both venous and arterial. The portal vein, carrying substances absorbed from the intestines, connects the liver with the gastrointestinal system. The oxygen-saturated blood from the aorta bathes the liver via the hepatic artery. The portal vein and artery branch through the liver in the form of a net and become small enough at their terminal ends to accommodate an actual mixture of arterial and venous blood. Blood which has bathed the liver reconvenes in the main hepatic veins and then enters the inferior vena cava to leave the abdomen and reach the right side of the heart.

The diverse functions performed by the liver are particularly essential to the human organism. The liver produces prothrombin, fibrinogen, insulin, and blood proteins; it manufactures and stores glucose and glycogen; it acts as the storehouse for iron, copper, vitamin A and vitamin D; it converts toxic into non-toxic substances; and when the heart fails to function properly, the liver expands to accommodate a larger quantity of blood. However, the function of the liver which is of concern to us here is the production of bile and its role in digestion.

Bile, which consists of 97% water and 3% various biochemical substances, is utilized in digestion, absorption, and elimination. From the liver, bile flows via the hepatic and cystic ducts into the gall bladder where, normally, it is stored. However, should the necessity arise, the liver may also assume this function.

The gall bladder, a long, narrow sequestration chamber lying midway between the intestine and the liver, is connected to the latter by the cystic duct, and to the intestine by the common duct. In the gall bladder, the thin bile receives mucus and becomes concentrated. At the time that it is required in the digestive act, the bile flows from the gall bladder, through the cystic duct, into the common duct and finally into the intestine. If more than the stored amount is needed, the liver will provide it directly through the hepatic and common ducts.

The liver offers a vast field for the researcher. Our concern will be with those studies discussing the effects of wine, or alcohol in equivalent dilutions, on the functions of the liver. Not so long ago, it was believed that wine was an important factor in the etiology of cirrhosis of the liver. However, recent studies show that normal consumption of wine has no such effect; and only if the liver has been previously damaged by malnutrition, or some other factor, might wine possibly contribute to the production of cirrhosis. Bollman (1938) studied dogs who had received alcohol with their daily rations for 2 years, and came to the conclusion that "alcohol in the presence of an adequate diet produces no demonstrable effect on the liver." A similar conclusion was reached by many others who investigated the etiology and production of cirrhosis of the liver. However, Jellinek (1940) reported that alcohol is a causative factor in the production of fatty liver, and that "The fatty liver constitutes a favorable condition for the development of the cirrhotic process when vitamin intake and carbohydrate intake are insufficient, or when the damaged liver is impaired in its assimilation, storage and utilization of vitamins." Klatskin (1951) in a paired feeding study on rats showed that alcohol increased the fat content of the liver even when the total caloric intake was not permitted to rise above that of the controls. These experiments suggest that alcohol may increase the choline requirement of the liver.

Most studies concerned with the effect of alcohol on the liver deal with either the etiology of cirrhosis of the liver, or damage to the liver ocurring in chronic alcoholism. Very few studies have been reported with regard to the effects of wine on the liver. One of the important studies was done in France by Loeper and coworkers, in 1929, who found that wines facilitate the assimilation of nitrogen and stimulate deamination by the liver; and that sweet wines and white table wines are more active in this respect than red table wines.

Data concerning the effect of wine on the gall bladder are indeed sparse. In one study (Da Cunha, 1939), it is reported that wine acts as a cholagogue when administered by duodenal tube but not when administered orally. In another study (Erdmann, 1953), it was found that the local effect of alcohol on the duodenal mucosa leads to reflex blocking of evacuation of the gall bladder. Recent experiments in the rat (Masquelier, 1964) showed that the intra-duodenal administration of the cinnamic derivatives of wine suspended in concentrated aqueous solution provoked an appreciable and constant increase in the flow of bile.

1794

Darwin, Erasmus ZOONOMIA, OR, THE LAWS OF ORGANIC LIFE. VOL. I, SEC. XXI: OF DRUNKENNESS. *London: J. Johnson. Reprinted in: Quart. J. Stud. Alc., 3:495–500, 1942.*

"Of Drunkenness," a chapter of the larger work, *Zoonomia,* is one of the earliest systematic attempts at explaining the physiologic effects of alcohol. These explanations are based entirely on conjecture. Referable to the liver, the author comments: "Hence in drunken people it generally happens, that the secretory vessels of the liver become first paralytic, and a torpor with consequent gallstones or schirrus of this viscus is induced with concomitant jaundice; otherwise it becomes inflamed in consequence of previous torpor, and this inflammation is frequently transferred to a more sensible part, which is associated with it, and produces the gout, or the rosy eruption of the face, or some other leprous eruption on the head, or arms, or legs." (p. 499)

1799

Sandford, William A FEW PRACTICAL REMARKS ON THE MEDICINAL EFFECTS OF WINE AND SPIRITS . . . *Worcester: J. Tymbs.*

"On the liver wine and spirits seem to exert a peculiar action—the biliary secretions are deranged; the bile necessarily becomes vitiated, its regular course interrupted, and its salutary uses lost to the constitution." (p. 64)

1814
Rush, Benjamin AN INQUIRY INTO THE EFFECTS OF ARDENT SPIRITS UPON THE HUMAN BODY AND MIND. *Brookfield: E. Merriam & Co., Eighth edition. (First edition, 1785) Reprinted in: Quart. J. Stud. Alc., 4:321–341, 1943.*

Written by a Philadelphia physician, this pamphlet represents the earliest American scientific work on inebriety. Though the value of his work is now obsolete scientifically, it contains acute medical observations and counsel. The author can find no benefit from the use of "ardent spirits" and suggests that these be replaced by cider, malt liquors, and wines. "These fermented liquors . . . are both cordial and nourishing." (p. 331) Among the "chronic effects of ardent spirits upon the body and mind," the author lists: "Obstructions of the liver. The fable of Prometheus, on whose liver a vulture was said to prey constantly, as a punishment for his stealing fire from heaven, was intended to illustrate the painful effects of ardent spirits upon that organ of the body." (p. 327)

1876
Richardson, (Sir) Benjamin W. ON ALCOHOL . . . *New York: The National Temperance Society and Publication House.*

"The effect of the alcohol upon the liver is upon the minute membranous capsular structure of the organ, upon which it acts to prevent the proper dialysis and free secretion. The organ at first becomes large from the distention of its vessels, the surcharge of fluid matter, and the thickening of tissue. After a time, there follow contraction of membrane and slow shrinking of the whole mass of the organ in its cellular parts. Then the shrunkened, hardened, roughened mass is said to be 'hobnailed,' a common but expressive term." (p. 160)

1886
Hirsch, August HANDBOOK OF GEOGRAPHICAL AND HISTORICAL PATHOLOGY. VOL. III. DISEASES OF ORGANS AND PARTS. *Translated by Charles Creighton from the second German edition. London: The New Sydenham Society.*

A study of the ecologic influence on and the geographic distribution of disease, in which the author ascribes the prevalence of hepatitis and abscess of the liver among the white population in the tropics to an inadequate diet and particularly to overindulgence in alcoholic drinks. These latter being readily available in the colonies, the incidence of alcoholism is very high among the troops. The author quotes Prof. Sachs as stating that "alcoholic drinks constitute in almost every case the direct etiological factor in the disease which is the subject of my observations [hepatitis]." He also cites Bryson's opinion that the recent decline in hepatitis is due to the better diet provided for the army, but particularly to the fact that the rum ration had been cut almost in half. The author further documents his personal observations by quotations from other writers on the subject.

1899

Boix, E. DE LA TOLERANCE ET DE LA RESISTANCE D'UN ORGANISME ROBUSTE ET DU FOIE EN PARTICULIER AUX BOISSONS ALCOOLIQUES. *Arch. Gén. Méd., 1:75–80.*

Written by the chief of the laboratories at the Faculty of Medicine, Paris, this article supports the thesis that alcohol alone is not responsible for the etiology of cirrhosis of the liver. To prove his point, the author gives a detailed case history of a man who had been a very heavy drinker for 30 years and though he had developed some dysfunction of the liver at the time of this writing, cirrhosis was not present.

1900

Mauriac, E. DEFENSE DU VIN AU TRIPLE POINT DE VUE: ECONOMIQUE, HYGIENIQUE ET THERAPEUTIQUE. *Xe Int'l. Congrès d'Hygiène et Demographie (Paris).*

"It is the abuse of alcohol which causes cirrhosis of the liver. It has been demonstrated that wine . . . plays no role in the production of this disease." (p. 183)

1906

Klopstock, F. ALKOHOLISMUS AND LEBERCIRRHOSE. *Virchow Arch. Path. Anat., 184:304–324.*

A report of experimental studies carried out at the Institute of Pathology, Berlin. Sections of liver from 25 patients with known, long-standing chronic alcoholism were analyzed. The results were compared with those of many other investigators in the field. It was concluded that chronic alcoholism might be a factor in predisposing the liver to cirrhosis but it is probably not responsible for its etiology.

Salant, W. THE EFFECT OF ALCOHOL ON THE SECRETION OF
BILE. *Amer. J. Physiol., 17:408–428.*

Report of experiments from the Department of Physiology
and Chemistry, Columbia University. The experiments were
carried out on dogs to whom various doses of alcohol were
given intravenously, and the bile collected at intervals of 15
minutes. "A comparison of the rates of secretion in alcoholized
and non-alcoholized dogs tended to show that alcohol interfered somewhat with the secretion of bile . . . On the other
hand, when alcohol was injected into the stomach or into the
intestines, there was a marked increase in the flow of bile,
and the solid elements were also increased absolutely and
relatively . . . [This increase] may be caused by secretin [which
may be produced when the augmented gastric secretions reach
the duodenum]. Secretin may excite not only the pancreas but
the liver as well." (pp. 426–428)

1908
Fischler, F. ÜBER EXPERIMENTELL-ERZEUGTE LEBERCIRRHOSE.
Deutsch. Arch. Klin. Med., 93:427–455.

After reviewing the literature, the author describes his investigations on dogs in whom he induced toxic cirrhosis of the
liver through the prolonged use of phosphorus and a mixture
of ethyl and amyl alcohol. He came to the conclusion that the
toxic cirrhoses of the liver were primarily a disturbance in the
parenchyma of the liver and that as long as the liver is capable
of handling intoxications, no disturbance in function occurs.

1914
Sbarboro, Andrea TEMPERANCE VS. PROHIBITION. IMPORTANT
LETTERS AND DATA FROM OUR AMERICAN CONSULS, THE CLERGY
AND OTHER EMINENT MEN. *San Francisco: H. S. Crocker Co;
Second edition.*

In the section dealing with "Opinions of Notable Foreign
Physicians on Wine," Dr. Tenedat, of the Academy of Mont-
pelier writes as follows:

"In the viticultural sections [of France], the workmen use
two quarts of wine per day. There are no alcoholics among
them and diseases of the liver are very rare. Many old men are
able to work until seventy-five and even eighty years." (p. 39)

1916
Bowers, Edwin F. ALCOHOL. ITS INFLUENCE ON MIND AND BODY.
New York: Edward J. Clode.

A virulent attack on alcohol in any form, at the beginning of which the author derives the word "alcohol" from the Arabic "al ghole"—evil spirit. On the liver, the author states: "Only recently has it been demonstrated that alcohol hinders the formation of glycogen in the liver, thus materially lessening the body's natural resistance to infection, and decidedly encouraging auto-intoxication from intestinal poisons." (p. 95)

1917

McJunkin, F. A. THE HUMAN AND ANIMAL LIVER AFTER ALCOHOL. *Arch. Intern. Med., 19:786–800.*

A report on 30 studies on the human liver performed at necropsy and some experimental studies on rabbits and guinea pigs designed to demonstrate the etiology of cirrhosis of the liver. In the necropsy studies, "alcohol is suggested as the causative agent by the history of these cases, but there is no further evidence to indicate that it injures the liver." In the animal studies alcohol produced no cirrhosis nor any "noteworthy lesion whatsoever of the liver cells . . . The so-called alcoholic cirrhosis is not produced directly by ethyl alcohol, that is, the liver is not injured by the alcohol carried to it through the blood or lymph." (pp. 799–800)

1931

Pousson VALEUR ALIMENTAIRE DU VIN. *Bull. Int. Vin., 4:44–48.*

An uncritical and often delicately naive analysis of the constituents of wine which are of nutritional value. On the liver, the author comments: "Glycerin, which in itself is one of the most precious nutritive substances, has, in addition, a very important effect on the functions of the liver." (p. 45)

1932

Sivo', R.; E. Egedy, and J. Erdös ALKOHOL UND LEBERCIRRHOSE. *Z. Ges. Exp. Med., 84:459–469.*

A report of experiments from the medical clinic of the University of Budapest in which an attempt was made to determine the cause of cirrhosis of the liver. It was found that in cirrhosis a marked increase in globulin is present, with a decrease in albumin. The authors believe that the increase in globulins in the livers of heavy drinkers is an indication of a predisposition to cirrhosis. In experiments on animals and on human beings, a single severe episode of alcoholic intoxication led to a transient increase in blood globulin.

1933
Carles, Jacques: PRECIS DE THERAPEUTIQUE APPLIQUEE. *Paris: G. Doin et Cie.*

"Wine taken in reasonable quantity has some rebuilding properties of the first order; but, taken in excess, even with the meal, it produces in the long run symptoms of alcoholic impregnation and creates hypertrophic cirrhosis." (p. 785)

MacNider, W. deB.: THE ACUTE DEGENERATIVE CHANGES AND THE CHANGES OF RECUPERATION OCCURRING IN THE LIVER FROM THE USE OF ETHYL ALCOHOL. A FUNCTIONAL AND PATHOLOGICAL STUDY. *J. Pharmacol. Exp. Ther., 49:100–116.*

The author reports an experimental investigation of the effects of toxic amounts of ethyl alcohol on the liver of the dog. Some of the observations were made after 12 hours of continuous intoxicating doses, and others after 24 hours of deep intoxication. The specific degrees of damage to the cells of the liver after withdrawal of the intoxicant were also noted. "The experiments indicate the ability of liver cells when reacting to the toxic action of large amounts of ethyl alcohol to undergo a severe edema from which they may recover without inaugurating a process of cell regeneration characterized by the formation of new cells." (p. 116)

1934
Moon, V. H. EXPERIMENTAL CIRRHOSIS IN RELATION TO HUMAN CIRRHOSIS. *Arch. Path., 18:381–424.*

A review article in which results from both clinical studies and experimental studies of cirrhosis of the liver as reported are carefully analyzed and evaluated. In summary, the author states: "Alcohol has been found to accentuate the injurious effects of bacteria, of phosphorus, of chloroform and of carbon tetrachloride on the animal liver. It is probable that alcohol may similarly [affect] the human liver. By virtue of this property alcohol may be an important contributory factor in the development of human cirrhosis . . . Its etiology will be found to be as variable as are the agents which, singly or in combinations, may cause chronic diffuse progressive inflammation of the liver." An extensive bibliography is appended.

1936
Boles, R. S., and J. H. Clark ROLE OF ALCOHOL IN CIRRHOSIS OF LIVER; CLINICAL AND PATHOLOGIC STUDY BASED ON 4,000 AUTOPSIES. *J.A.M.A., 107:1200–1203.*

A statistical analysis of 4,000 autopsies. The authors make an effort to correlate cirrhosis of the liver to other pathologic conditions. From the results it was concluded that "alcohol cannot be regarded as a specific factor in the etiology of cirrhosis. As the lesion defined as portal cirrhosis occurs under influences unassociated with alcohol, we suggest abandonment of the term 'alcoholic cirrhosis.' "

Dieulafé, L., and Miquel SUR LA PATHOGENIE DE LA CIRRHOSE DE LAENNEC. *IIIe Congrès Nat'l. Méd. Amis des Vins de France, Dijon, pp. 151–160.*

A report of clinical case histories diagnosed as Laennec's cirrhosis. A thorough study of the individual past histories was undertaken in order to attempt and establish the etiology of this disease. Among the alcoholic beverages, it was found that cocktails, alcohols of undefined origin, beer and then wines were the worst offenders—in that order. With regard to wine in the etiology of Laennec's cirrhosis, the investigators studied the types of wine consumed and came to the conclusion that they were always inferior wines, grown in bad soils and from mediocre vines, made with poor vinification techniques. The resulting wine, the authors believe, has certain damaging chemical characteristics, a ferric taste, and a very high volatile acidity.

1938

Bollman, J. L. SOME EXPERIMENTAL OBSERVATIONS PERTINENT TO THE TREATMENT OF HEPATIC DISEASE. *Ann. Intern. Med., 12:2–5.*

"We have given alcohol to the stage of definite intoxication to dogs twice daily for more than two years. Those animals which took a well-balanced diet during this time showed no gross or microscopic hepatic abnormalities . . . Alcohol in the presence of an adequate diet produces no demonstrable effect on the liver, but when food is withheld or when diets predominantly fat are given with the alcohol, the liver rapidly becomes fatty. With a fat diet that would produce fatty livers in dogs in from six to eight weeks, the addition of alcohol causes the liver to become fatty in two or three days. It is quite probable that alcohol may in a like manner increase the susceptibility of the liver to other toxic agents." (p. 3)

1939

Connor, C. L. THE ETIOLOGY AND PATHOGENESIS OF ALCOHOLIC

CIRRHOSIS OF THE LIVER. *J.A.M.A., 112:387–389.*

A paper presented at the 89th Anniversary Session of the American Medical Association, in which the author defines the various types of cirrhosis (toxic, biliary, pigmentary and fatty) and discusses the etiology of alcoholic cirrhosis. The discussion is based on clinical studies and observations at autopsy. The author feels that the following combinations will eventually result in alcoholic cirrhosis of the liver: 1) starvation, or partial starvation, plus large amounts of alcohol habitually; 2) diet restricted to protein plus fat, and alcohol; 3) diet containing an insufficient amount of carbohydrates and vitamins, plus large amount of alcohol habitually; and 4) alternating periods of well-balanced diet with periods of severe alcoholism and insufficient diet.

daCunha-Franco, R., and C. Santos VINO EN LA COLECISTO-
GRAFIA. *Dia Méd., 6:131–132.*

The authors describe wine as a cholagogue and in support of this statement they quote the authority of Loeper, Michaux and deSèze. The latter authors probed the duodenum with an Einhorn tube and used red and white wine instead of magnesium sulfate in the experiment of Meltzer-Lyon. The introduction of wine produced an abundant flow of bile (up to 10 times the quantity of wine introduced) greater than that produced by magnesium sulfate. With 20 ml. of wine, 190 ml. of bile was obtained, and with magnesium sulfate only 100 ml. White wines appeared to be more active cholagogues than red wines. According to the authors, the effect of wine as a cholagogue depends upon its content of magnesium salts, potassium tartrate, alcohol and amino acids, as well as its pH value. Loeper and coworkers believe that wine affects the cells and biliary function as well as the gall bladder itself in this reflex action which stimulates secretion and is dependent upon the effect of the wine directly on the cells.

Tests by DaCunha-Franco and Santos failed to confirm the report of Loeper, et al. The authors used eggs as the control nutrient, and found that wine neither excites nor inhibits vesicular motility. The fact that Loeper and deSèze used a tube to deposit the wine in the duodenum, while daCunha-Franco and Santos administered the wine orally is held to account for the fact that the wine remained pure in one study, while in the latter study it reached the duodenum mixed with the contents of the stomach. The authors of this article conclude that wine taken in the ordinary manner does not empty the gall bladder.

Hall, E. M., and W. A. Morgan PROGRESSIVE ALCOHOLIC CIR-
RHOSIS. A CLINICAL AND PATHOLOGICAL STUDY OF SIXTY-EIGHT
CASES. *Arch. Path., 27:672–690.*

This report consists of a clinico-pathological study of 68
cases of subacute or progressive alcoholic cirrhosis. Only one
of the patients denied having used alcohol, and at least 80%
were chronic alcoholics. "Alcoholism was the outstanding,
most common clinical factor in this group of cases . . . We believe the term 'alcoholic cirrhosis' has a firm basis in etiology."
(pp. 689–690)

1940

Boles, R. S., and R. S. Crew OBSERVATIONS ON CHRONIC ALCO-
HOLISM AND CIRRHOSIS OF THE LIVER. *Quart. J. Stud. Alc., 1:
464–471.*

A report on 210 cases of cirrhosis of the liver from observations at autopsy and clinical histories of patients with the
purpose in mind of determining the relation, if any, between
cirrhosis of the liver and chronic alcoholism. In summarizing
their findings, the authors state: ". . . an alcoholic history was
obtained in only 68, or 32.4 per cent [of the cases studied]. In
the portal type of cirrhosis, ordinarily alluded to as 'alcoholic
cirrhosis,' a history of alcoholism was obtained in 40 [out of
a total of 88 cases] or 45.5 per cent . . . While it is recognized
that alcohol may play a role, and perhaps a predominating
role, in a certain indeterminate number of cases of cirrhosis,
it should be equally well recognized that in a great number of
cases, factors other than alcohol would appear to be responsible for the cirrhosis." (pp. 470–471).

Connor, C. L. CIRRHOSIS OF THE LIVER. *Quart. J. Stud. Alc.,
1:95–102.*

An article in which the historical data and the more recent
experimental data are reviewed, and in conclusion the author
stresses the fact "that there are many different kinds of cirrhoses of the liver caused by many substances . . . and that
recognition of this fact is elementary and fundamental before
a study of this group of diseases can be started; . . ." (p. 101)

Jellinek, E. M., and N. Jolliffe EFFECTS OF ALCOHOL ON THE
INDIVIDUAL. REVIEW OF THE LITERATURE OF 1939. *Quart. J.
Stud. Alc., 1:110–181.*

"The possibility of direct causation of cirrhosis by alcohol is entirely dismissed. On the other hand, the production of fatty liver is being definitely attributed to prolonged use of alcohol. The fatty liver constitutes a favorable condition for the development of the cirrhotic process when vitamin intake and carbohydrate intake are insufficient, or when the damaged liver is impaired in its assimilation, storage, and utilization of vitamins." (p. 132)

Jolliffe, N. VITAMIN DEFICIENCIES AND LIVER CIRRHOSIS IN ALCOHOLISM. INTRODUCTION AND PART I. *Quart. J. Stud. Alc., 1: 517–557.*

After reviewing recent literature pertaining to alcoholic polyneuropathy, its pathology, and etiology, the author presents some conclusions to be drawn from these data. "It should be clearly stated that, although these diseases do unquestionably develop as a direct result of nutritional deficiency, it is the ingestion of too much alcohol that is responsible for the nutritional deficiency." (p. 518)

Newman, H. W.; W. Van Winkle, Jr.; N. K. Kennedy, and M. C. Morton COMPARATIVE EFFECTS OF PROPYLENE GLYCOL, OTHER GLYCOLS AND ALCOHOL ON THE LIVER DIRECTLY. *J. Pharmacol. Exp. Ther., 68:194–200.*

Experimental report from the Department of Pharmacology, Stanford University (California), in which the effects of propylene glycol on the isolated liver of the cat were compared with those of ethyl alcohol and some other glycols. The results showed that "1. Propylene glycol decreased the oxygen consumption and carbon dioxide production of the perfused isolated cat's liver, but increased the glycogen of the liver and the lactic acid content of the blood and decreased the utilization of dextrose by the liver. 2. Addition of insulin to the perfusion with propylene glycol caused a further depression of the oxygen consumption of the liver, prevented the increase of blood lactic acid, and hastened the utilization of the glycol, in agreement with a reputedly similar action of insulin on alcohol." (p. 199)

1941

Cates, H. B. ACUTE HEPATITIS OF ALCOHOLISM: A CLINICAL AND LABORATORY STUDY. *Ann. Intern. Med., 15:244–250.*

Report of case histories on 25 alcoholic patients admitted to the Los Angeles County Hospital. Most of the subjects had been on an alcoholic spree for more than two weeks, some for as long as six weeks. All 25 exhibited abnormal bromsulfalein tests and were "regarded as being cases of hepatitis unrecognized clinically. A certain number of this group [were considered to] have a progressive liver deterioration leading eventually to Laennec's cirrhosis." (pp. 249–250)

Cates, H. B. RELATION OF LIVER FUNCTION TO CIRRHOSIS OF THE LIVER AND TO ALCOHOLISM. *Arch. Intern. Med., 67:383–398.*

A clinico-pathological study of 42 patients diagnosed as having cirrhosis of the liver. An effort was made to correlate the results of liver function tests with anatomic changes in the liver. The tests used were: analysis of serum proteins, hippuric acid, bromsulfalein, and cholesterol; biopsy of the liver was carried out on all patients, and in addition all but one patient were examined peritoneoscopically. Alcohol was considered as a contributing factor to the cirrhosis of the liver in at least 28 patients, 17 of whom "suffered from acute alcoholism." The author considers the bromsulfalein test to be the most valuable indicator of dysfunction of the liver.

Jolliffe, N. VITAMIN DEFICIENCIES AND LIVER CIRRHOSIS IN ALCOHOLISM. PART II. CIRCULATORY DISTURBANCES. PART III. PELLAGRA. *Quart. J. Stud. Alc., 1:727–750.*
    and
Jolliffe, N.; H. Wortis, and M. H. Stein *Ibid.* PART IV. THE WERNICKE SYNDROME. PART V. NICOTINIC ACID DEFICIENCY ENCEPHALOPATHY. PART VI. ENCEPHALOPATHIES WITH POSSIBLE NUTRITIONAL INVOLVEMENTS. *Quart. J. Stud. Alc., 2:73–97.*
    and
Jolliffe, N., and E. M. Jellinek *Ibid.* PART VII. CIRRHOSIS OF THE LIVER. *Quart. J. Stud. Alc., 2:544–583.*

"Its [alcohol's] direct toxic action in producing pellagra is very questionable. 'Alcoholic' pellagra may then be considered to be a disease resulting from the deficiency of vitamin B complex, predominantly nicotinic acid, occurring in alcohol addicts." (Vol. 1, p. 747) "Although the syndrome [Wernicke's] is most usually associated with chronic alcoholism, there is good evidence that alcohol, per se, is not responsible for the clinical picture." (Vol. 2, p. 85)

Mochizuki, N. CLINICAL STUDY OF CHRONIC HEPATOPATHY. REPORT 6. HEPATITIC FUNCTIONS OF HABITUAL DRINKERS AND SOME PERSONS SUFFERING FROM CHRONIC OPIUMALKALIDTOXICOSIS.

(Japanese text) J. Orient. Med., 34:49. (Abstract in: Quart. J. Stud. Alc., 2:838, 1942.)

"The hepatic functions of 11 habitual drinkers who had been using alcoholic beverages for 8 to 35 years were investigated. In 7 of the 11 patients the liver disturbances could be recognized morphologically as well as functionally. In 3 there were only slight functional disturbances. Even in the presence of severe hepatic disturbances in habitual drinkers 'it was corroborated that they could become convalescent or even recover in a relatively short period by means of both abstinence from alcohol and some hyperfunctional treatments of the liver, provided that such detriments had not already been deteriorated into cirrhosis.' " (Quoted verbatim from Quart. J. Stud. Alc.)

1942

Beazell, J. M.; A. L. Berman; V. H. Hough, and A. C. Ivy THE EFFECT OF ACUTE ALCOHOLIC INTOXICATION ON HEPATIC FUNCTIONS. *Amer. J. Dig. Dis., 9:82–85.*

An experimental study on 10 normal, healthy males reported as "occasional drinkers." The subjects received dinner at 6 p.m. and were told to begin consuming whiskey with soda or gingerale at 8 p.m. and drink ad libitum for the next 4 hours, thereby completing the experiment at midnight. One-half hour later, blood samplings began, and liver function tests were performed at 10 a.m. the following morning. On the average, the men consumed 2–3 cc. of alcohol per kilogram of body weight. The correlation of intake of alcohol with symptoms was poor. The stage of intoxication reached in this study was without ill-effects on the liver.

Fleming, R. G., and A. M. Snell PORTAL CIRRHOSIS WITH ASCITES: AN ANALYSIS OF 200 CASES WITH SPECIAL REFERENCE TO PROGNOSIS AND TREATMENT. *Amer. J. Dig. Dis., 9:115–120.*

A clinical analysis of 200 cases of portal cirrhosis of the liver with ascites. In 42.5% alcohol was found to be an etiologic factor. In analyzing the treatment of these patients, the authors state that excellent results were obtained with "a high carbohydrate, high vegetable protein diet and large doses of vitamins." (p. 120)

Jellinek, E. M., editor ALCOHOL ADDICTION AND CHRONIC ALCOHOLISM. EFFECTS OF ALCOHOL ON THE INDIVIDUAL. A CRITICAL EXPOSITION OF PRESENT KNOWLEDGE. VOLUME I. *New Haven: Yale University Press.*

As the title implies, the book presents a critical review of the literature on the subject of alcoholism. Among the contributors to the volume are Drs. Bowman, Jolliffe, Wortis, Stein, and Lolli. The topics reviewed are: Alcohol Addiction and Its Treatment, and Alcoholic Mental Disorders, by Bowman and Jellinek; Vitamin Deficiencies in Chronic Alcoholism, by Jolliffe; Alcoholic Encephalopathies and Nutrition, by Jolliffe, Wortis and Stein; Marchiafava's Disease, by Lolli; and, Cirrhosis of the Liver, by Jolliffe and Jellinek. Referable to cirrhosis of the liver, it is stated: "While the association between inebriety and cirrhosis of the liver is definitely established and a direct causation through alcohol is ruled out, none of the numerous etiologic theories of indirect causation can be accepted at present as sufficiently documented. On the other hand, diversity of the etiologies is not to be taken as a sign of confusion or of lack of knowledge, since most of these theories are not mutually exclusive but can be integrated into a common theory." (p. 309)

Marsh, F. B. DISEASES OF THE LIVER; CLINICAL FEATURES; LIVER FUNCTION TESTS; AND TREATMENT. *Virginia Med. Monthly, 69:70–77.*

An article reviewing diseases of the liver in which it is pointed out that fatty livers frequently occur in users of large amounts of alcohol. This change, it is stated, represents the early stage of alcoholic-type cirrhosis. The author lists the following stages in the development of alcoholic cirrhosis of the liver: consumption of large amounts of alcohol, loss of appetite, limited food and inadequate vitamin intake—all of these favor development of fatty liver which then undergoes fibrosis. The treatment recommended is an adequate diet high in protein and rich in vitamin B-complex.

1943

Boles, R. S. ALCOHOL AND CIRRHOSIS OF THE LIVER. *Southern Med. J., 36:353–358. (Abstract in: Quart. J. Stud. Alc., 4:345, 1943.)*

A review of recent findings concerning the role of alcohol in cirrhosis of the liver. The author concludes that it is incorrect to use the terms "alcoholic cirrhosis" and "portal cirrhosis" synonymously, since the latter condition frequently occurs without alcohol as an element of its etiology.

Kirschbaum, J. D., and N. Shure ALCOHOLIC CIRRHOSIS OF THE LIVER; A CLINICAL AND PATHOLOGIC STUDY OF 356 FATAL CASES

SELECTED FROM 12,267 NECROPSIES. *J. Lab. Clin. Med., 28: 721–731.*

A statistical study performed at the Cook County Hospital, Chicago. Cirrhosis of the liver was diagnosed in 356 instances (2.83%); of these latter, cirrhosis was the primary cause of death in 184. The age groups 41 to 60 for males and 31 to 50 for females, contributed the largest number of cases. Among the 356 instances, 144 had a definite history of chronic alcoholism, but a clinical history was not uniformly available for all subjects of the series.

1944

György, P. EXPERIMENTAL HEPATIC INJURY. *Amer. J. Clin. Path., 14:67–88.*

A paper presented at the 22nd Annual Meeting of the American Society of Clinical Pathology, in which the author reviews recent work on experimental hepatic injury. "Low intake of protein combined with insufficient supply of the vitamin B-complex (including choline) is a prominent feature of the daily diet of persons addicted to alcohol and is in good agreement with the contributing conditions of dietary cirrhosis in rats . . . The postulate of a specific injurious effect of alcohol becomes superfluous just as it does in conditions of pellagra or beriberi of alcoholics." (p. 84) The author then makes several suggestions for the prevention and treatment of hepatic injury in man.

1945

Graham, G. S., Jr. PORTAL CIRRHOSIS: ITS ETIOLOGY, DIAGNOSIS AND TREATMENT. *Miss. Doctor, 22:195–201. (Abstract in: Quart. J. Stud. Alc., 7:314, 1946.)*

The author discusses the relationship between alcoholism and cirrhosis of the liver in view of recent findings. The primary change caused by excessive use of alcohol is fatty infiltration of the liver which, the author believes, is the result of toxic action of alcohol on tissue oxidation, insufficient and vitamin deficient diets resulting from chronic excessive use of alcohol, and the toxic nature of alcohol together with associated infections.

1946

Halonen, P. I., and N. Saksela LIVER CIRRHOSIS IN FINLAND. *Ann. Med. Intern. Fenn., 35:7–33.*

A statistical study of 134 cases of liver cirrhosis found at necropsy spanning the years 1920–1945. These cases represented 1.8% of all necropsies. Among them, 29 were known alcoholics, 10 moderate users, and 19 had claimed to be abstainers. No histories with reference to alcohol consumption were available on the remaining 76 instances. The male to female ratio was 0.7:1. It is tentatively concluded that alcohol probably increases the incidence of cirrhosis.

1947

Ashworth, C. T. PRODUCTION OF FATTY INFILTRATION OF LIVER IN RATS BY ALCOHOL IN SPITE OF ADEQUATE DIET. *Proc. Soc. Exp. Biol. Med., 66:382–385.*

A report of experiments in three groups of rats, one receiving low casein diet plus alcohol, the second high casein diet plus alcohol, and the third low casein diet alone. As controls, rats receiving a high casein diet alone were used. Fatty infiltration of the liver occurred in all animals receiving the low casein diet alone. The high casein diet alone did not cause fatty infiltration. The author therefore concluded that alcohol exerts an effect which permits accumulation of fat within the liver cells and that this effect operates separately from that of extrinsic deficiency of lipotropic factors.

Boles, R. S.; R. S. Crew, and W. Dunbar ALCOHOLIC CIRRHOSIS. *J.A.M.A., 134:670–673.*

A statistical study of 3,637 autopsies, among which 142 instances of cirrhosis of the liver were found. The male to female ratio was 1.25:1. The ratio between the white and the negro race was 3.89:1. In 64 of the 142 instances, a history of alcohol use was obtained, and among these 50 had a history of definite alcoholism; total abstinence was noted in 14. In 50 instances a clinical diagnosis of cirrhosis had been made and among these 33 had a positive history of alcoholism. "Such figures tend to prove that alcohol causation be absolved from contributing its part to the causation of cirrhosis in an indeterminate number of persons." (p. 672)

1948

Barborka, Clifford J. TREATMENT BY DIET. *Philadelphia: J. B. Lippincott Company, Fifth edition. (First edition, 1934)*

A standard textbook in the field of nutrition, dealing with diet in health, the application of diet therapy, diet in disease, and routine hospital diets. Alcoholic beverages are discussed primarily in relation to diseases of the liver. "It is quite evident then that alcohol alone cannot be considered responsible for cirrhosis of the liver. According to Connor, the nutritional errors of the alcoholic, who would rather drink than eat, are the basis of liver damage. On the other hand, it is doubtful whether any alcoholic on an adequate diet will develop cirrhosis." (pp. 496–497)

Chaikoff, I. L.; C. Entenman; T. Gillman, and C. L. Connor PATHOLOGIC REACTIONS IN THE LIVER AND KIDNEYS OF DOGS FED ALCOHOL WHILE MAINTAINED ON A HIGH PROTEIN DIET. *Arch. Path.*, *45:435–446*.

A report of an experimental study in which dogs were given large quantities of alcohol (a 22.5% solution in amounts up to 240 cc. per day) while being maintained on a high protein diet, adequate in all respects. Erratic feeding habits developed. The results showed severe hepatic and renal injury. However, the authors could not determine whether these pathologic changes were due to the alcohol or the associated malnutrition.

Chalmers, T. C.; T. L. Murphy, and E. B. Taft THE INCIDENCE, CHARACTER AND COURSE OF LIVER DISEASE IN CHRONIC ALCO- HOLICS, AS DETERMINED BY NEEDLE BIOPSY. *J. Clin. Invest.*, *27: 528–529*.

A statistical and pathological report on 24 patients ad- mitted to the hospital with incipient or active delirium tre- mens. Biopsies of the liver were performed within a few days of admission and all showed pathologic changes. Among the 24 subjects, 12 were steady drinkers and 12 intermittent drinkers who stopped work and took hardly any nourishment while on an alcoholic bout. The 12 steady drinkers showed more fibrosis and necrosis than the 12 intermittent drinkers.

Haggie, M. ALCOHOL AND CIRRHOSIS OF THE LIVER. *London Hosp. Gaz.*, *51:69–72*.

A statistical study of 408 instances of portal cirrhoses found among 23,949 necropsies. A correlation between the degree of alcoholism and the incidence of cirrhosis was attempted.

Sanes, S.; W. H. C. Chapple, and R. C. Bahn NEEDLE BIOPSIES OF THE LIVER IN ALCOHOLIC PATIENTS. *Proc. N.Y. State Assn. Public Health Lab.*, *28:56–58*.

A report of findings in 54 alcoholic patients admitted to the E. J. Meyer Memorial Hospital (Buffalo) in a state of acute intoxication and in whom a needle biopsy was performed.

Among the 54 subjects, 25 showed fatty liver, 18 showed cirrhosis, 3 were "unclassified pathology" and 8 were reported to possess normal livers. The histories for most of these cases showed long-standing deficient diets and alcoholism, but the author did not draw any conclusions as to which of these circumstances was responsible for the condition of the liver.

1949
Best, C. H.; W. S. Hartroft; C. C. Lucas, and J. H. Ridout
LIVER DAMAGE PRODUCED BY FEEDING ALCOHOL OR SUGAR AND ITS PREVENTION BY CHOLINE. *Brit. Med. J., 2:1001–1006.*

A report of paired feeding experiments on rats, one group receiving 15% alcohol instead of water, another an isocaloric quantity of sucrose in lieu of the alcohol solution, and other groups receiving various lipotropic supplements to their diets. "The results suggest that an imbalance between calorie intake and supply of accessory food factors is the cause of the liver lesions: the extra calorie intake induces a specific deficiency when the basal diet is marginal with respect to any one vitamin. Alcohol or sugar, when taken in excess, supplants choline-containing foodstuffs and at the same time, by increasing the calorie intake, augments the demand for lipotropic agents . . ., 'the conclusion may be drawn that the hepatic changes associated with the ingestion of pure ethyl alcohol in this experiment were due to an induced choline deficiency." (p. 1005)

Brit. Med. J. CIRRHOSIS OF THE LIVER. *(Summary of Proceedings of the 117th Annual Meeting, Section of Med.), 2:166–167.*

A discussion of the material presented with regard to cirrhosis of the liver. Dr. M. H. K. Haggie (London) was of the opinion that "alcohol was a factor in the cause of cirrhosis; but alcoholics often did not eat, and were therefore deficient in the necessary protective factors." Dr. E. R. Cullinan (London) "did not believe that acute hepatitis frequently progressed to cirrhosis." Dr. H. Steinitz (Israel) stated that though there were many kinds of liver damage in Israel, "true cirrhosis of the liver with portal hypertension, haematosis, and ascites was very rare." He did not know the cause, but stated that "there was almost no drunkenness in Israel or in the Arab population of Palestine." (p. 167)

Hobson, W. ALCOHOL AND CIRRHOSIS OF THE LIVER. *Brit. Med. J. (Correspondence), 2:1228–1229.*

A letter reporting a statistical study on mortality in a population sample which included innkeepers, hotelkeepers and bartenders. The author found the mortality among innkeepers to be 11.5 times higher than in the population as a whole, and among bartenders six times higher. These figures correspond with an earlier study dealing with the effect of sugar and alcohol on fat deposits, and the author poses the question that "if the suggestion of adding choline to alcoholic drinks is to be taken seriously, why not include sweets at the same time?" (p. 1228)

Voegtlin, W. L.; W. R. Broz; W. E. Tupper, and M. M. Robinson LIVER FUNCTION IN CHRONIC ALCOHOLIC PATIENTS. II. CORRELATION BETWEEN ELEMENTS OF HISTORY AND PRESENCE OF LIVER DYSFUNCTION AS INDICATED BY LABORATORY TESTS. *Gastroenterology, 13:391–400.*

In 300 alcoholic patients dysfunction of the liver was more severe among the steady than among the periodic drinkers, regardless of the type of beverage—whiskey, bonded liquor, beer or wine. Dysfunction was more common in those who enjoyed an increased tolerance to alcohol than in those with decreased tolerance, and in those who had experienced "blackouts." The study shows no clear-cut indication for predicting liver dysfunction in alcoholics, but indicates that liver dysfunction induced by alcohol is temporary and reversible.

1950

Cachera, R.; M. Lamotte, and S. Lamotte-Barrillon L'EVOLUTION DES STEATOSES ALCOOLIQUES DU FOIE CONTROLLEE PAR PONCTIONS-BIOPSIES. *Bull. Soc. Méd. Hôp., (Paris) 66:292–302.* *(Abstract in: Quart. J. Stud. Alc., 11:663.)*

Thirty-five patients with steatosis and six with cirrhosis of the liver were studied by means of the needle-biopsy technique and the rate of development or reduction of steatosis was shown to be variable. A regression of steatosis occurred in 13 of the patients, two of whom had reduced their intake of alcohol. In ten patients who continued the excessive use of alcohol, the steatosis remained unchanged.

Olsen, A. Y. A STUDY OF DIETARY FACTORS, ALCOHOLIC CONSUMPTION AND LABORATORY FINDINGS IN 100 PATIENTS WITH HEPATIC CIRRHOSIS AND 200 NON-CIRRHOSIS CONTROLS. *Amer. J. Med. Sci., 220:477–484.*

A study concerning the dietary and alcoholic histories of

100 cirrhotic patients and 200 non-cirrhotic subjects who acted as controls. Seventy-eight per cent of the patients in the cirrhotic group were "heavy" and 14 per cent were "moderate" drinkers. The author discusses alcohol and nutritional deficiencies as a factor in the etiology of cirrhosis of the liver. "Our findings seem further to substantiate evidence both experimental and clinical, which suggests that portal cirrhosis has as its basis a multiple nutritional deficiency, chiefly of protein and the B-complex foodstuffs and that alcohol is probably a significant indirect causative factor insofar as it causes faulty dietary habits." (p. 483)

Tsunoda, K. STUDIES ON THE ANTITOXIC FUNCTION OF THE LIVER. II. ON THE ANTITOXIC FUNCTION OF POTORS AND HABITUAL DRINKERS. *Tohoku J. Exp. Med., 52:299–305.*

Report of a clinical study from the Tohoku University Medical Clinic, on 29 habitual drinkers who demonstrated overt or clinical findings of disturbance of the liver. The results showed that "livers of potors who are resistant to much quantity of spirits are considered to possess such antitoxic function as is superior to that of normal men." (p. 304)

Vansteen-Huyse, F. LEBER EN CHRONISCH ALCOHOLISME. *Belg. Tijdschr. Geneesk. 6:734–738. (Abstract in Quart. J. Stud. Alc., 12:137–138, 1951.)*

A review of the recent literature on the relationship between alcoholism and diseases of the liver. The author discusses the data and concludes that alcohol does not cause cirrhosis of the liver but does cause fatty degeneration—thus creating a predisposing factor to cirrhosis. The same effects may be obtained from a diet lacking in lipotropic factors provided the sugar content is high.

Voegtlin, W. L.; W. E. Tupper, and M. M. Robinson LIVER FUNCTION IN CHRONIC ALCOHOLIC PATIENTS. III. CORRELATION BETWEEN THE PRESENCE OF LIVER DYSFUNCTION AS INDICATED BY LABORATORY AND OBJECTIVE FINDINGS ON EXAMINATION. *Gastroenterology, 14:485–490.*

A follow-up study on a group of 300 chronic alcoholic patients in an attempt to correlate the degree of dysfunction of the liver with the objective findings at physical examination. "On the basis of the data presented it may be stated that the objective findings in chronic alcoholics do not suggest that such patients characteristically suffer from portal cirrhosis." (p. 490)

Welin, G. NEEDLE BIOPSY AND LIVER FUNCTION IN EARLIER STAGES OF FATTY CIRRHOSIS OF THE LIVER. *Acta Med. Scand., Supplement 246:260–267.*

Clinical and biopsy study of 13 patients admitting alcoholism and showing some degree of liver involvement. All the patients were males between the ages of 38 to 59 and in some of them a history of imbibition of 1 liter of distilled liquor daily was obtained. Needle function tests as well as needle biopsy studies were carried out in all subjects. The findings support the assumption made by Connor (1938–1939) that long standing, fatty infiltration of the liver results in more severe disease of that organ. "Whether the alcohol as a toxic agent or the deficient diet, which undoubtedly is often connected with severe alcoholism, is the cause of the progressive fibrosis is a question which cannot be answered on the basis of this investigation." (p. 265)

1951

Del Greco, F., and R. Maffei LA RESPONSABILITÀ DELL'ALCOOL NELL'ETIOLOGIA DELLA CIRROSI EPATICA DI MORGAGNI-LAENNEC. *Gaz. Int. Med. Chir. (Napoli), 55:813–820. (Abstract in: Quart. J. Stud. Alc., 13:315, 1952.)*

Comparative dietary and drinking study on two groups of 100 patients each, one composed of cirrhotic and the other non-cirrhotic subjects. In the cirrhotic group, 80 were users of wine and among these 29 drank between 2–4 liters daily, and 3 about 1½ liters daily. In the non-cirrhotic group, 70 were users of wine—3 drinking over 2 liters daily and 8 about 1½ liters daily. After reviewing the dietary habits of these two groups, the authors conclude that "alcohol is not a specific etiological factor in liver cirrhosis, but that it causes malnutrition in the habitual drinker."

Klatskin, G.; H. M. Gewin, and W. A. Krehl EFFECTS OF PROLONGED ALCOHOL INGESTION ON THE LIVER OF THE RAT UNDER CONDITIONS OF CONTROLLED ADEQUATE DIETARY INTAKE. *Yale J. Biol. Med., 23:317–331.*

An experimental report on 6 groups of pair-fed rats receiving the same basal diet. In one group, alcohol *ad libitum* was given; a second group received no alcohol; a third group received an isocaloric supplement of sucrose instead of alcohol; a fourth group received the basal diet plus alcohol but the total caloric intake was the same as the group receiving the basal diet and no alcohol; and the fifth group received the basal diet *ad libitum* with no supplements. Comparable groups of animals were sacrificed at 117 days and at 180 days. The livers were examined chemically and histologically. The average concentration of total lipids was within normal limits in all groups, but the range and distribution differed significantly in the alcohol-fed groups. "The fact that alcohol increased the fat content of the liver . . . even when the total caloric intake was not permitted to rise above that of pair-fed controls is strong evidence against the hypothesis that alcohol, like carbohydrate, increases the demand for choline by raising the caloric intake. Rather these experiments suggest that alcohol may increase the choline requirement in some other way, possibly by blocking its action in the liver, by altering its absorption from the intestinal tract, or by altering its rate of endogenous synthesis." (p. 330)

1952

Eger, W. DAS ZENTRALE UND PERIPHERE FUNKTIONSFELD DES LEBERLÄPPCHENS UNTER DER EINWIRKUNG VON ÄTHYL- UND METHYL-ALKOHOL. *Med. Mschr., 6:363–367. (Abstract in: Quart. J. Stud. Alc., 15:333, 1954.)*

An experimental study on rats and guinea pigs fasted for 3 to 4 days and then given 1 cc. of 48% alcohol per 100 gram of body weight through a stomach tube. The animals were sacrificed 8 hours after administration of alcohol. The livers were examined for glycogen and fat. In rats, the glycogen was greatly diminished and fat greatly increased; in guinea pigs, these findings were not so marked.

Lebon, J.; M. Fabregoule, and R. Eisenbeth LES CIRRHOSES NON-ALCOOLIQUES DU MUSULMAN NORDAFRICAIN. *Presse Méd.* 60:1528.

The cirrhosis of the liver which occurs in the non-alcohol-imbibing Moslems is caused by malnutrition; and in addition, malaria may be of etiological significance. Among the Moslems who are not religious and do not practice abstinence, there also occurs "alcoholic" cirrhosis.

Sepulveda, B.; E. Rojas-Natera, and L. Landa LA ETIOLOGIA DE LA CIRRHOSIS DEL HIGADO TIPO LAENNEC. *Rev. Invest. Clin. Mex., 4:321–339.*

A statistical and clinical investigation of 150 cases of cirrhosis of the liver. Among the subjects, 132 consumed more than 50 cc. of alcoholic beverages daily, and 18 consumed more than 100 cc. daily. The dietary intake was inadequate in 140 subjects, while in 10 the diet could be considered adequate. It is concluded that alcoholism without malnutrition does not cause cirrhosis of the liver, and if abnormalities of the liver occur they are usually reversible.

Uhry, P., and A. Morel-Maroger SUR 34 OBSERVATIONS DE CIRRHOSE SUIVIES EN 1951. *Presse Méd. 60:883–885. (Abstract in: Quart. J. Stud. Alc., 14:327, 1953.)*

A statistical and clinical study of 34 patients suffering from cirrhosis of the liver seen during the year 1951. Among these, 29 were alcoholics who had consumed an average of 2–3 liters of wine daily. After treatment, improvement occurred in 11; there was no change in 10, 10 had died, and in 3 the condition became aggravated. The author draws no conclusions, except to state that "it is salutary for them [the patients] to see others die, for then they become fearful, stop drinking and recover."

1953

Erdmann, W. D., and H. F. Henne DER EINFLUSS VON GENUSS-GIFTEN AUF DIE GALLENENTLEERUNG. *Klin. Wschr., 31:989–992.*

The effects of coffee, nicotine, alcohol, and benzedrine on gall bladder evacuation in the dog was studied. With regard to alcohol it was found that the local effect of alcohol on the duodenal mucosa leads to impairment of the emptying mechanism of the gall bladder.

Girard, M.; M. Plauchu, and C. Loisy LES CIRRHOSES. ESSAI DE CLASSIFICATION. *J. Méd. Lyon, 34:71–93.*

An essay in which the authors recommend a new classification system of cirrhoses: perilobular cirrhosis (divided into toxic cirrhosis, post-steatotic cirrhosis, viral, infectious, pigmentary, and zoo-parasitic cirrhosis); mesenchymatous cirrhosis; and cardiac cirrhosis. With regard to the role of alcohol in cirrhosis, the authors state: "Steatosis and alcoholic cirrhosis are not caused by the direct toxic action of the alcohol on the liver, but are the result of dietary disturbances caused by the alcohol. Steatosis and alcoholic cirrhosis are nutritional diseases." (p. 82)

Klatskin, G. THE ROLE OF ALCOHOL IN THE PATHOGENESIS OF CIRRHOSIS. *Yale J. Biol. Med., 26:23–37.*

A review of literature of experimental findings with reference to alcohol and cirrhosis from which the author concludes that "while dietary factors play an important role in the pathogenesis of alcoholic cirrhosis, a great deal remains to be learned about the complex interrelationships between alcohol consumption, dietary deficiencies, and alterations in the structure of the liver." (p. 35)

Leevy, C. M.; I. Patrylo, and W. Doody HEPATIC ABNORMALITIES IN ALCOHOLICS WITH DELIRIUM TREMENS. *Quart. J. Stud. Alc., 14:568–575.*

A report from the Jersey City Medical Center of histological studies of the liver correlated with clinical and biochemical findings in 66 alcoholic patients with delirium tremens. The results of this study "did not provide a clue to the encountered histology." The authors are of the opinion that "hepatic abnormalities in delirium tremens appear to be due to dietary inadequacies . . . The degree of alcoholism and severity of cerebral symptoms could not be correlated with hepatic abnormalities." (p. 574)

Wanscher, O. EXPERIMENTAL PORTAL CIRRHOSIS. PATHOGENESIS AND RELATION TO ADMINISTRATION OF ALCOHOL. *Acta Path. Microbiol. Scand., 32:348–354.*

A report of experimental work from The Vitamin Laboratory and Institute of Pathology, Sundby Hospital, Copenhagen. Thirty-seven rats were kept on a diet low in cystine and methionine supplemented with varying quantities of cystine and choline; 20 of these rats received in addition, 20% alcohol as their fluid, and 17 rats received only water. The results showed development of fatty liver with necroses; the addition of choline to the diet prevented fatty degeneration but not the formation of necroses; portal cirrhosis did not occur, and administration of alcohol did not influence results. "According to present-day knowledge, the fatty liver of the alcoholic is not the result of the alcohol intoxication in itself, but of insufficient nutrition, particularly a too-low intake of proteins . . . Since alcohol is, moreover, a destructive poison to the enzymatic processes in the alimentary tract, it is reasonable to assume that the splitting as well as the absorption of proteins is deficient in the alcoholic. When also combined with the scanty intake of the important proteins, this gives rise to fatty degeneration of the liver." (p. 353)

Zieve, L., and E. Hill. INFLUENCE OF ALCOHOL CONSUMPTION

ON HEPATIC FUNCTION IN HEALTHY GAINFULLY EMPLOYED MEN. *J. Lab. Clin. Med., 42:705–712.*

A clinical study of 744 presumably healthy men, half of whom had had viral hepatitis 4–6 years prior to the study; all were gainfully employed, and their dietary habits were satisfactory. The consumption of alcoholic beverages varied: 14 consumed approximately one-fifth gallon of distilled liquor per day; 80 consumed between 6–8 oz. per day; 387 consumed between 1–3 oz. per day, and 262 had only an occasional drink or none at all. Eleven different tests of liver function were performed on each patient. From the analysis of laboratory data it is clear "there is no prominent relationship between alcohol consumption and hepatic function in men whose nutrition and health are normal. Relatively large amounts of alcohol may be consumed without evident abnormality of hepatic function tests." (pp. 709–710)

1954

Martens, S. ALKOHOLISM OCH LEVERSJUKDOM. *Nord. Med., 51: 439–444. (Abstract in: Quart. J. Stud. Alc., 16:360, 1955.)*

"Needle aspiration biopsies of the liver were performed in 32 hospitalized adult males with the clinical diagnosis of alcoholism. Fatty degeneration of the liver was present in 20 of them: slight in 9, moderate in 3 and pronounced in 8. Its presence was positively correlated with the severity of alcoholism, with signs of lowered resistance to alcohol, and with the presence of nervous and mental conditions caused by alcoholism. It occurred less frequently in spree drinkers than in steady drinkers." (Quoted verbatim from Quart. J. Stud. Alc.)

Phillips, G. B., and C. S. Davidson ACUTE HEPATIC INSUFFICIENCY OF THE CHRONIC ALCOHOLIC. CLINICAL AND PATHOLOGIC STUDY. *Arch. Intern. Med., 94:585–603.*

Detailed histologic and functional findings in 56 patients with acute hepatic impairment and alcoholism. Alcoholics may have a typical hepatic lesion, rarely, if ever, seen in nonalcoholics, which may result from direct or indirect effect of alcohol on the liver. It is characterized by "hyaline degeneration, liver cell necrosis and parenchymal disorganization, which is distinct from the fatty lesion and is usually responsible for the . . . acute severe liver impairment, which may improve slowly but often leads to fatal hepatic coma." (pp. 601–602)

1955

Allert, M. L. ALKOHOLISMUS UND LEBERCIRRHOSE. *Med. Klin.,*

50:1815–1816.

A statistical study of 106 cases of cirrhosis of the liver found at necropsies performed during 1950–1955. Among these cases, only 11 presented a definite history of alcoholism. The clinical impression that increasingly newer patients with cirrhosis have a history of alcoholism is confirmed.

Serianni, E.; G. Lolli, and M. Venturini THE EFFECTS OF SOLID FOOD AND OF ALCOHOLIC BEVERAGES, ESPECIALLY WINE, ON THE EXCRETION OF HIPPURIC ACID. *Quart. J. Stud. Alc., 16:67–85, 1955.*

Experiments showed that wine with a meal caused a marked increase in the excretion of hippuric acid.

Therefore, in using the hippuric acid test for a measurement of liver function, one must have in mind the effects which ingestible substances, including wine and other alcoholic beverages, may have upon its excretion, and which may necessitate a correction in the calculated results of the test.

1956

Mallov, S., and J. L. Bloch ROLE OF HYPOPHYSICS AND ADRENALS IN FATTY INFILTRATION OF LIVER RESULTING FROM ACUTE ETHANOL INTOXICATION. *Amer. J. Physiol., 184:29–34.*

The authors demonstrate that ethanol intoxication may cause the mobilization of fat from depots to the liver, and that pituitary and adrenal cortical hormones are involved in the mechanism of mobilization.

1957

Lefft, H. H. SOME NUTRITIONAL AND THERAPEUTIC ASPECTS OF WINE AND COGNAC. *Int. Rec. Med., 170:361–368.*

Referable to the liver, the author states: "The notion that alcohol plays a major role in the etiology of hepatic cirrhosis has never been demonstrated conclusively. It has been thoroughly reported that this disease is one of deficiency, and is seen both in the livers of alcoholics and in subjects who do not drink at all. In fact, Jolliffe has commented that excessive ingestion of sweet carbonated beverages is as likely to produce cirrhosis as is chronic alcoholism." (p. 362)

1958

Di Luzio, N. R. EFFECT OF ACUTE ETHANOL INTOXICATION ON LIVER AND PLASMA FRACTIONS IN THE RAT. *Amer. J. Physiol., 194:453–456.*

The fatty liver (expressed as elevated plasma neutral fat)

following acute ethanol intoxication is discussed with particular references to its possible hepatotoxic action. There was noted an initial increase in plasma cholesterol, followed by a rise in phosphatides and somewhat later an elevation in neutral fat. It is suggested that the plasma lactescence noted in chronic alcoholics is probably due to acute pancreatitis associated with alcoholism.

1960

Isselbacher, K. J., and E. A. McCarthy EFFECTS OF ALCOHOL ON THE LIVER; MECHANISM OF THE IMPAIRED GALACTOSE UTILIZATION. *Amer. J. Clin. Invest., 39:999–1000.*

Alcohol inhibits galactose metabolism in the liver by producing increased cellular levels of DPNH (Diphosphopyridine nucleotide) which inhibits the key enzyme in galactose metabolism (uridine diphogalactose-4-ipimerase). These results serve to emphasize the importance of cellular concentration of pyridine nucleotides in the overall regulation of carbohydrate metabolism.

1962

Lieber, C. S., and C. S. Davidson SOME METABOLIC EFFECTS OF ETHYL ALCOHOL. *Amer. J. Med., 33:319–327.*

A good review article devoted to some aspects of the biochemistry and physiology of the metabolism of alcohol, particularly involving the liver.

1964

Masquelier, J., and J. Laparra ACTION CHOLERETIQUE DES CONSTITUANTS CINNAMIQUES DU VIN. *Bull. Soc. Pharm. Bordeaux, 103:121–122.*

The cinnamic constituents of red wine were extracted by ethyl acetate, purified, and placed in concentrated aqueous solution. In the rat carrying a ductus choledochus fistula, the intraduodenal administration of this solution provoked an appreciable and constant increase in the flow of bile.

1965

Dajani, R. M.; L. Ghandur-Mnaymneh; M. Harrison, and T. Nassar THE UTILIZATION OF ETHANOL. III. LIVER CHANGES INDUCED BY ALCOHOL. *J. Nutr., 86:29–36.*

Marquardt, P., and H. W. J. Werringloer TOXICITY OF WINE. *Food Cosmet. Toxic., 3:803–810.*

Marquardt draws attention to the potential toxicity of wines and attributes this to the histamine content which appears as a result of improper hygienic control evidenced during the process of vinification.

Tygstrup, N.; K. Winkler, and F. Lundquist THE MECHANISM OF THE FRUCTOSE EFFECT ON THE ETHANOL METABOLISM OF THE HUMAN LIVER. *J. Clin. Invest., 44:817–830.*

Fructose given intravenously almost doubles the splanchnic ethanol uptake and acetate output. When fructose or ethanol is given alone, it has no appreciable effect on the splanchnic blood flow and oxygen uptake, but when they are given together, the blood flow is increased by about 30% and the oxygen uptake by about 60%. During infusion of ethanol the splanchnic uptake of fructose is increased on the average by about 0.6 millimol per minutes, compared with fructose infusion alone, and a corresponding amount of polyol (mainly sorbitol) is encountered in the hepatic veins. The splanchnic output of lactate and pyruvate is reduced to one-third during ethanol-fructose infusion compared with fructose infusion alone. In this process fructose is reduced to sorbitol which presumably contributes to the fructose effect.

1966

Brohult, J., and H. Reichard LIVER DAMAGE IN HEALTHY SUBJECTS AFTER INTAKE OF ALCOHOL. PRELIMINARY REPORT. *Nord. Med., 75:128–130.*

The author comments upon the elevated level of ornithine-carbamoyl-transferase (O.C.T.) in the blood serum as a specific sign of liver damage. The O.C.T. activity in serum rose in 8 healthy volunteers when 200–300 g. of ethanol as distilled spirits was given. The 2 subjects who were given an identical amount of ethanol as wine did not exhibit a rise in O.C.T. level.

1967

Leuschner, F., and A. Leuschner VERGLEICHENDE TIEREXPERIMENTELLE UNTERSUCHUNGEN MIT WEINEN AUS HYBRIDEN-UND EUROPÄERREBEN. *Arzneimittelforschung, 17:59–66.*

The authors compare the physiological and anatomical effects on the livers of rats given wines made of hybrid grapes and wines made of pure *Vitis vinifera* origin. They discuss in detail the differential effects of these wines concerning experimentally induced fatty degeneration of the liver. The physiology of altered-hepatic metabolism under the conditions of the experiment are thoroughly discussed.

Lieber, C. S.: CHRONIC ALCOHOLIC HEPATIC INJURY IN EXPERI-MENTAL ANIMALS AND MAN: BIOCHEMICAL PATHWAYS AND NU-TRITIONAL FACTORS. *Fed. Proc., 26:1443–1448.*

In the discussion of this paper, J. Cueto presents his views regarding a like experiment and he summarizes: "We have found no evidence that ethanol in the rhesus monkey in a dose level of 3 g/kg. per day has a significant effect on liver structure or function, when protein and choline are given to supplement the diet." (p. 1448)

Porta, E. A.; W. S. Hartroft; C. L. A. Gomez-Dumm, and O. R. Koch DIETARY FACTORS IN THE PROGRESSION AND REGRES-SION OF HEPATIC ALTERATIONS ASSOCIATED WITH EXPERIMENT-AL CHRONIC ALCOHOLISM. *Fed. Proc., 26:1449–1457.*

The authors make a valuable contribution to the controver-sial subject of altered hepatic function and chronic alcohol-ism in this paper on experimentally-altered metabolism and liver disease in the rat. The protocol is carefully devised, de-signed, and implemented by adequate analysis, both biochemi-cal and cytological. They conclude that "a direct hepatotoxic action of alcohol" in their experiments on the rat "is an un-likely one." In man, they offer the suggestion that "the asso-ciation . . . between chronic consumption of spirits and liver injury is a result of induced or relative multi-factoral dietary deficiency," and their experiences have persuaded them "to abandon terms such as alcoholic fatty liver and alcoholic cirrhosis," in favor of "alcohol-conditioned injury." (p. 1457)

1968
Gomez-Dumm, C. L. A.; E. A. Porta; W. S. Hartroft, and O. R. Koch A NEW EXPERIMENTAL APPROACH IN THE STUDY OF CHRONIC ALCOHOLISM. II. EFFECTS OF HIGH ALCOHOL INTAKE IN RATS FED DIETS OF VARIOUS ADEQUACIES. *Lab. Invest., 18: 365–378.*

The authors conclude that "the type of diet is more impor-tant than the amount of alcohol as a determinant of at least two of the most frequently associated hepatic changes, tri-glyceride accumulation and mitochondrial deformation." (p. 365) Severe hepatic lesions were not found even in those rats which were fed only pretzels together with high amounts of al-

cohol for six weeks, and which, consequently, failed to grow
and suffered a 60% mortality rate.

Koch, O. R.; E. A. Porta, and W. S. Hartroft A NEW EXPERI-
MENTAL APPROACH IN THE STUDY OF CHRONIC ALCOHOLISM. III.
ROLE OF ALCOHOL VERSUS SUCROSE OR FAT-DERIVED CALORIES
IN HEPATIC DAMAGE. *Lab. Invest., 18:379–386.*

The authors reported that a diet generously supplemented
with vitamins, lipotropes, and salts fed to rats along with
high amounts of alcohol prevented almost completely any
hepatic fatty changes and proved to be more effective in the
maintenance of the normal integrity of the liver than did the
same diet fed to the control rats in which either sucrose, fat,
or a combined mixture of sucrose, fat, and protein isocalorically replaced the alcohol.

Lelbach, W. K. LIVER DAMAGE FROM DIFFERENT ALCOHOLIC
DRINKS. *German Med. Monthly, 13:31–39.*

A discussion of the alcoholic contents of different alcoholic
beverages in terms of the "extent of liver damage." The author
recognizes that the presence of "additives and contaminants
play a secondary role." The significance of the paper is limited by the author's consideration of ethanol as the important
factor, without a satisfactory explanation of the many other
ingredients which we know are contained in alcoholic beverages, natural and manufactured.

Porta, E. A., and C. L. A. Gomez-Dumm A NEW EXPERIMENT-
AL APPROACH IN THE STUDY OF CHRONIC ALCOHOLISM. I. EF-
FECTS OF HIGH ALCOHOL INTAKE IN RATS FED A COMMERCIAL
LABORATORY DIET. *Lab. Invest., 18:352–364.*

The authors conclude that "our findings add emphasis to
the importance of induced nutritional alterations in the pathogenesis of hepatic lesions associated with chronic alcoholism
rather than to any theoretically direct hepatotoxin action of
alcohol." (p. 352)

**Porta, E. A.; O. R. Koch; C. L. A. Gomez-Dumm, and W. S.
Hartroft** EFFECTS OF DIETARY PROTEIN ON THE LIVER OF RATS
IN EXPERIMENTAL CHRONIC ALCOHOLISM. *J. Nutr., 94:437–446.*

The lipotropic effect of dietary protein was tested in rats
fed for 16 weeks a liquid diet in which 40% of the calories
were provided by alcohol and 25% by an amino acid mixture.

Controls received a comparable diet in which sucrose isocalorically replaced the alcohol. The livers were examined and levels of hepatic triglycerides, cholesterol and phospho-lipids were determined at 4-week intervals for 16 weeks. In the early stages (4–8 weeks) of the experiment, the alcohol-consuming rats developed more extensive fatty liver than did controls. The accumulation of fat which was only moderate in degree proved to be transient because it later disappeared (12–16 weeks). But fat in livers of control rats did not disappear. Instead, it progressively accumulated during the entire 16-week period. Some mitochondrial alterations and a few Mallory bodies were also observed at the early stages in rats consuming alcohol. However, these ultra-structural changes sharply regressed so that by the end of the experiment livers from both groups were almost indistinguishable and almost normal (aside from the fat in livers of the carbohydrate controls). These data support the concept that even if alcohol has any postulated hepatotoxic effects on the livers of rats, it can be modified by manipulation of the accompanying diet.

Rubin, E., and C. S. Lieber ALCOHOL-INDUCED HEPATIC INJURY IN NONALCOHOLIC VOLUNTEERS. *New Eng. J. Med., 278:869–876.*

The authors conclude on controversial evidence that alcohol is a hepatotoxic agent, independent of nutritional factors. They present materials obtained by biopsy to support their hypothesis. However, the fact that their experimental data do not adequately establish incontrovertible scientific evidence of their beliefs is brought out and discussed in an editorial entitled "Is Alcohol Hepatotoxic?" which appears in the same issue of the journal (on pp. 905–906).

EFFECTS ON ABNORMAL FUNCTIONS

In surveying the literature referrable to the effects of wine on the malfunctioning liver, it becomes evident that a reasonable and definite conclusion must await further observation and experimentation. The majority of investigations are concerned basically with the effects of alcohol, rather than wine, on cirrhosis of the liver. There is very little pertinent information available on the effects of wine on jaundice, acute hepatitis, fatty liver, amyloid disease, and neoplasms. A clinical and statistical study of soldiers who had had either infectious or serum hepatitis and who had resumed drinking alcoholic beverages showed no more evidence of liver damage than abstainers who had had the disease.

The literature regarding the effects of wine on cirrhosis indicates that wine can be of assistance mainly for its ability to stimulate appetite and to act as a tranquilizer (Summerskill, 1957). An interesting observation in this area, and one which needs further confirmation, is offered by Carbone (1957), who reported that the addition of wine to the carefully controlled diet of cirrhotic patients under hospital supervision appeared to improve the clinical status of the patient and, inferentially, the immediate status of the liver.

The major pathological conditions of the gall bladder—dyskinesia, cholelithiasis, acute and chronic cholecystitis, and cholangiohepatitis—seem to have escaped pertinent observation. The review of the literature discloses no studies directly referrable to the effect of wine on disorders of the gall bladder.

1930

Rosenthal, S. M. SOME EFFECTS OF ALCOHOL UPON NORMAL AND DAMAGED LIVER. *J. Pharmacol. Exp. Ther., 38:291–301.*

Experimental studies in which 98% alcohol, diluted to 33%, was administered by stomach tube to dogs in doses of 2 cc. per kilogram of body weight. The effect of alcohol on the normal liver and on the liver previously damaged by chloroform or carbontetrachloride was studied. In both the normal and pre-damaged liver, there was slight impairment of function which returned to normal after 24 hours.

1933

Eylaud, J. M., and R. Marcard VIN AU POINT DE VUE HYGIEN-IQUE. *Bull. Int. Vin, 6:90–99.*

The authors give a recipe for onion wine to be used in the treatment of cirrhosis: "Onion wine for cirrhosis: raw onion 200 cc.; white liquid honey 100 cc.; white wine 700 cc.; three glasses of this wine daily." (p. 94)

1937

Desgeorges LE VIN CHEZ LE ENTERO-HEPATIQUES. *IVe Congrès Nat'l Méd. Amis des Vins de France, Alger, pp. 76–81.*

"If there is reason to prohibit wine to patients with severe liver diseases, there is no reason to let those with minor hepatic disturbances suffer from this prohibition. The entero-hepatic patients in particular will find in wine not only an agreeable and strengthening beverage, but to a certain extent a veritable remedy." (pp. 80–81)

1938
Connor, C. L., and I. L. Chaikoff PRODUCTION OF CIRRHOSIS IN FATTY LIVERS WITH ALCOHOL. *Proc. Soc. Exp. Biol. Med., 39: 356–359.*

A report of experiments on 16 dogs in an effort to produce cirrhosis within the fatty liver. The dogs received a high fat diet for the first 30–35 days, followed by the administration of 10 cc. of 22.5% alcohol per kilogram of body weight and low fat intake for 4–7 days alternated with a similar period of feeding fats. The results showed excessively fatty livers in all animals, some with intrahepatic obstruction; there was atrophy of liver cells at the periphery with hyaline degeneration; 4 of the 16 animals showed moderate, but definite cirrhosis.

1941
Lillie, R. D.; F. S. Daft, and W. H. Sebrell, Jr. CIRRHOSIS OF THE LIVER IN RATS ON A DEFICIENT DIET AND THE EFFECT OF ALCOHOL. *Public Health Rep., 56:1255–1258.*

A report on experimental work, from the Division of Pathology and Chemotherapy, National Institute of Health, undertaken to test the effect of the ingestion of alcohol on rats receiving a diet known to have certain deficiencies. Four groups of rats were used, all receiving variously deficient diets and two groups receiving water *ad libitum,* while the other two groups received approximately 20% alcohol *ad libitum.* The pathologic liver changes which occurred seemed more severe on the average, where the alcohol was substituted for water. "In these particular experiments, it would appear that alcohol gives an additional insult to liver tissue injured by dietary deficiency." (p. 1257)

Patek, A. J., Jr., and J. Post TREATMENT OF CIRRHOSIS OF THE LIVER BY A NUTRITIOUS DIET AND SUPPLEMENTS RICH IN VITAMIN B COMPLEX. *J. Clin. Invest., 20:481–505.*

A clinical study dealing with 54 patients suffering from cirrhosis of the liver and being treated with a well-balanced diet and supplements rich in vitamin B complex is reported. Of the patients, 20 recovered, 12 improved, and 22 failed to show any change. In order to study the effect of alcohol further, the authors selected 4 among the recovered patients to whom, in addition to the nutritious diet and vitamin B complex sup-

plements, they administered 9 oz. of 40% alcohol daily for
6, 10, 14, and 18 months respectively. There was no recur-
rence of symptoms; the bromsulfalein, the Takata-Ara and
the serum protein tests showed no pertinent changes.

1942

Lowry, J. V.; L. L. Ashburn; F. S. Daft, and W. H. Sebrell EF-
FECT OF ALCOHOL IN EXPERIMENTAL LIVER CIRRHOSIS. *Quart.
J. Stud. Alc., 3:168–175.*

A report of experiments carried out under the auspices of
the United States Public Health Service. Albino rats, paired
in litter mates of the same sex, were given a low protein, low
choline diet plus a daily vitamin B-complex supplement. A
second series of experiments, with the rats paired as above,
was carried out and the animals were allowed to eat *ad libitum*, but one rat of each pair drank water while its mate received a 20% solution of alcohol as its source of fluid. The
results showed that "although hepatic cirrhosis can be consistently produced in rats by dietary means without the use
of alcohol, the process in a given length of time is usually
more severe when alcohol is substituted for drinking water
. . . The influence of alcohol on the development of liver
cirrhosis probably involves a much more complex mechanism
than direct toxicity." It was found that, "Alcohol increases the
severity of the liver cirrhosis produced in rats with a deficient diet." (p. 174–175)

Snell, A. M. CHANGING CONCEPTIONS OF PORTAL CIRRHOSIS.
*Penn. Med. J., 45:337–344. (Abstract in: Quart. J. Stud. Alc.,
3:146, 1943.)*

A review of recent experimental work in the production of
cirrhosis of the liver in animals by deficient diets. The author
concludes that alcohol acting on a liver impaired by nutritional defect may produce cirrhosis of the liver, while the same
amount of alcohol would do little permanent harm to the liver
in a normal state.

1948

Volwiler, W.; C. M. Jones, and T. B. Mallory CRITERIA FOR THE
MEASUREMENT OF RESULTS OF TREATMENT IN FATTY CIRRHO-
SIS. *Gastroenterology, 11:164–182.*

It was noted "that a moderate alcohol intake will not prevent satisfactory repair of liver damage in fatty cirrhosis provided the dietary intake is ample and well balanced." (p. 181)

1949
Gardner, H. T.; R. A. Rovelstad; D. J. Moore; F. A. Streitfeld, and M. Knowlton HEPATITIS AMONG AMERICAN OCCUPATION TROOPS IN GERMANY: A FOLLOW-UP STUDY WITH PARTICULAR REFERENCE TO INTERIM ALCOHOL AND PHYSICAL ACTIVITY. *Ann. Intern. Med. 30:1009–1019.*

A clinical and statistical follow-up study of 114 soldiers who were re-examined 6 to 12 months after discharge from the Hepatitis Center, Medical Department, U.S. Army European Command in Germany. The subjects, 19 to 36 years old, had been hospitalized initially for infectious hepatitis or serum hepatitis for an average of 62 days. On re-examination the only residual finding was a slight deviation in the thymol turbidity test. Residua were found in 12 of 28 heavy drinkers, 11 of 23 moderate drinkers, 7 of 35 light drinkers and 11 of 26 abstainers. Subjects who drank one quart of wine, six glasses of beer, or six oz. of distilled spirits daily for 6 to 12 months after the attack of acute hepatitis showed no more evidence of liver damage than did the total abstainers.

1952
Sirnes, T. B. THE BLOOD ALCOHOL CURVE IN ZONAL NECROSIS OF THE LIVER. *Quart. J. Stud. Alc., 13:189–195.*

A report of experimental work, from the Department of Pharmacology, University of Oslo, in which the influence of different types of liver injury on rate of alcohol oxidation was investigated. Lesions of the liver were induced in 2 groups of rats—with carbon tetrachloride in one and phosphorus in olive oil in the other. When the lesions were thought to be maximal, all rats received 2 g. of a 20% solution of ethyl alcohol per kilogram of body weight. The alcohol was injected intravenously into the femoral vein. The first blood samples were taken 30–70 minutes after injection and then at one or two hour intervals up to 2 hours. Following sacrifice, the liver tissue was examined histologically. A third group of normal rats was used as controls. In the group receiving carbon-tetrachloride the rate of alcohol oxidation differed little from that of the normal group. Oxidation was much slower in the group receiving phosphorus. "These experimental results seem to indicate that the central portion of the liver lobule does not participate so actively in the oxidation of ethyl alcohol as does the peripheral portion." (p. 195)

1953

Sirnes, T. B. VOLUNTARY CONSUMPTION OF ALCOHOL IN RATS WITH CIRRHOSIS OF THE LIVER. A PRELIMINARY REPORT. *Quart. J. Stud. Alc., 14:3–18.*

A preliminary report on experimental work carried out at the Department of Pharmacology, University of Oslo. Cirrhosis of the liver was produced in 20 albino rats by subcutaneous injections of carbon-tetrachloride. In the course of the first 3 months, 6 rats died; the remaining 14 rats were maintained on an identical diet and were given a choice of either water or 20% alcohol solution. Ten normal rats were used as controls. Blood and urine samples were analyzed for alcohol content, and the amount of each fluid consumed was measured daily. It was found that, "The voluntary intake of alcohol . . . in rats with cirrhosis of the liver, was approximately four times as great as in a control group with normal livers." (p. 17) The author postulates that this may be due to the effect of alcohol on the thiamine requirements, namely that alcohol has a sparing effect on the thiamine requirement.

1954

Danopoulos, E.; K. Maratos, and J. Logothetopoulos STUDIES ON THE ALCOHOL'S METABOLISM IN PATIENTS WITH ATROPHIC LIVER CIRRHOSIS. *Acta Med. Scand., 148:485–492.*

Clinical studies on 10 in-patients (7 males, 3 females) with liver cirrhosis. After a 12-hour fast, each patient received 0.60 cc. of alcohol per kilogram of body weight. The alcohol content of the blood and ascitic fluid was measured at intervals of one-half hour and then every hour for four hours. In five cases an equivalent amount of alcohol was injected into the peritoneal cavity at least seven days after the first experiment. The results, in this instance, indicated that metabolism of alcohol in patients with atrophic cirrhosis of the liver is definitely impaired although the configuration of the curves is usually normal. This, the authors believe, is due to the fact "that a certain quantity of alcohol diffuses into the ascitic fluid, wherefrom it is absorbed by the peritoneum and brought back to the circulating blood and through it to the whole organism, to be burned." (p. 492) This same phenomenon, the authors believe, is responsible "for the appearance of intoxication signs that are milder than those expected from the amount of alcohol administered." (p. 492)

1956

Strauss, M. B.; W. H. Birchard, and L. Saxon CORRECTION OF IMPAIRED WATER EXCRETION IN CIRRHOSIS OF THE LIVER BY ALCOHOL INGESTION OR EXPANSION OF EXTRACELLULAR FLUID VOLUME: THE ROLE OF THE ANTI-DIURETIC HORMONE. *Trans. Ass. Amer. Physicians, 69:222–228.*

A report of an experimental study of three groups of patients with hepatic cirrhosis and ascites, in whom the excretion of urine was markedly depressed. The patients were studied following ingestion of alcohol (one-half pint of 100 proof Bourbon whiskey diluted with water *ad libitum* and taken within about one hour) and after the hypotonic expansion of their extracellular fluid volume. Following the ingestion of alcohol, there was "augmented flow of urine of a decreased concentration [which] speaks for a previous release of anti-diuretic hormone in response to a non-osmotic stimulus in these patients. The temporal relationship between the height of urinary alcohol concentration and maximum diuresis suggests that there is no delay in the removal of circulating antidiuretic hormone from the blood of these patients. Evidence for the role of a contracted *effective* extracellular fluid volume as the non-osmotic stimulus for ADH release could not be elicited in most of these patients, although this may have been the result of experimental design.

Patients with hepatic cirrhosis and ascites, not as severely ill, whose renal excretory capacity for water was only *moderately* limited achieved virtually normal diuresis concomitant with an increased renal sodium excretion when their extracellular fluid volume was expanded.

It was concluded that increased antidiuretic hormone release may play a role in the *markedly* impaired water excretion of certain patients with hepatic cirrhosis. The inability to excrete sodium, or some factor associated therewith, possibly conditioned by a contraction of the *effective* extracellular fluid volume, appears to be an important factor in the *moderately* impaired water excretion encountered in many patients with hepatic cirrhosis." (p. 228)

1957

Carbone, J.; V. Sborov; R. Fanska, and K. Ringgold THE EFFECT OF WINE IN DECOMPENSATED HEPATIC CIRRHOSIS. *J. Clin. Invest., 36:878.*

Clinical experiments in which 1 liter of red table wine was administered to 5 chronic alcoholic patients suffering from severe cirrhosis of the liver. The patients were kept on diets controlled in calories and protein values. Liver biopsy studies showed marked clearing of the fatty and cellular infiltrations characteristic of this disease.

Summerskill, W. H. J.; S. J. Wolfe, and C. S. Davidson RESPONSE TO ALCOHOL IN CHRONIC ALCOHOLICS WITH LIVER DISEASE. CLINICAL, PATHOLOGICAL AND METABOLIC CHANGES. *Lancet, 272:335–340.*

A clinical study of alcoholic patients with malnutrition and liver disease. The patients were kept on a well-balanced diet and after a control period were given 90 to 120 ml. of ethyl alcohol in fruit juice, divided into 6 daily doses, for 10–32 days. It was found that the alcohol had no adverse effect; in two, the livers decreased in size and in all patients with peripheral neuritis, improvement in muscle power and gait occurred. "The most striking clinical effects of alcohol were the increased appetite and the euphoria that immediately followed its addition to the regimen. These facts suggest that small doses of alcohol should be given therapeutically to alcoholics with liver disease, because the anorexia which often complicates their management may be due to abstention." (p. 339)

1962

Di Luzio, N. R. COMPARATIVE STUDY OF THE EFFECT OF ALCOHOLIC BEVERAGES ON THE DEVELOPMENT OF THE ACUTE ETHANOL-INDUCED FATTY LIVER. *Quart. J. Stud. Alc., 23:557–561.*

It is concluded that the various congeners present in commercial alcoholic beverages (blended whiskey, bourbon, cognac, gin, scotch, vodka) given by oral intubation in a single dose (i.e., 6 g. per kg. of body weight as a 50% solution) neither increased nor decreased the severity of acute fatty liver which appears to be specifically due to the influence of ethanol on hepatic triglyceride metabolism.

CONTRAINDICATIONS

As any old soldier who has had jaundice knows, medical opinion tends to proscribe the use of alcoholic beverages in this disorder. But the literature on the subject is meager. Lolli and Rubin have reported that obstructive jaundice induced in rats did cause a marked decrease in the disappearance of alcohol from the blood.

As previously noted, dietary insufficiency perhaps is the major cause of cirrhosis. Excessive amounts of any alcoholic beverage ingested while a person is on an inadequate diet may well induce cirrhosis. Indirect evidence would seem to indicate that wine or any other alcoholic beverage should be prohibited in cases of cirrhosis, except when the patient, under hospital conditions, is being maintained on a 3,000-calories diet rich in proteins and B vitamins. In the latter instance, wine may be included in order to stimulate appetite.

In the early part of this century, some of the attacks on alcohol included its proscription because of damage to the liver, but these are based mainly on opinion as opposed to fact.

While there is no experimental evidence to indicate that wine or other alcoholic beverage should be avoided by a patient suffering from any one of the major gall bladder disorders, clinical experience has indicated this to be the wisest approach. After cholecystectomy, however, there is no reason to proscribe wine except for special and individual causes.

1917

Labbé, Marcel REGIMES ALIMENTAIRES. *Paris: J. B. Baillière et fils, Second edition.*

On the liver, the author states: "Wine is to be avoided in hepatic affections." (p. 458)

1943

Lolli, G., and M. Rubin THE RATE OF DISAPPEARANCE OF ALCO-HOL FROM THE BLOOD IN OBSTRUCTIVE JAUNDICE. *Quart. J. Stud. Alc., 4:183–186.*

A report of experimental studies from the Laboratory of Applied Physiology, Yale University. Obstructive jaundice was induced by surgical ligation of the common duct in 14 rats; another 14 rats without obstructive jaundice served as controls. Twenty-four hours after the surgical procedure, all rats received 3 g. per kilogram of body weight of absolute alcohol in 50% solutions. Blood samples were taken from the heart at 2-, 4-, and 6-hour intervals, and the alcohol concentration in the blood determined. The results showed that the presence of obstructive jaundice causes a marked decrease in the rate of disappearance of alcohol from the blood.

1957

Stokes, J. F., and M. L. Rosenheim TREATMENT IN DIFFUSE LIVER DISEASE. *Brit. Med. Bull., 13:142–145.*

"Another symptom that may follow hepatitis is alcohol intolerance . . . The treatment is abstention and the intolerance disappears, as a rule, in 18 months. This intolerance is probably the basis for the common advice to avoid all alcohol for six months in convalescence. In our view an occasional glass of wine or sherry is not contra-indicated." (p. 142)

1960

Ferguson, M., and M. Marie ALCOHOL IN CLINICAL MEDICINE. *GP, 21:108–114.*

"It is common practice to prohibit liquor for periods of months to years in patients recovering from viral hepatitis. Despite this, there has been no controlled study to indicate that alcohol *per se* has any toxic effects on the normal or post-hepatic liver . . . It is interesting to note that the recent international symposium on viral hepatitis does not even allude to the question of alcohol following hepatitis. The well-known animal studies which indicated alcohol itself is hepatotoxic have been adequately refuted by less well-known but more complete laboratory studies." (p. 111)

6

The Effects of Wine and its Constituents on the Functions and Disorders of the Pancreas

EFFECTS ON NORMAL FUNCTIONS

Lying in an S-shaped curve formed by the stomach and the duodenum, the pancreas is an elongate pyriform structure. The right end—its head—is connected by a duct to the duodenum. The pancreas contains glands that secrete digestive enzymes which are delivered into the duodenum, and isolated nests of cells known as the islets of Langerhans which secrete insulin. The latter function of the pancreas does not concern us at this time; it is its role as a producer of enzymes that is our current preoccupation.

The pancreas begins its activity when secretin (a hormone produced in the duodenum and jejunum), elaborated during digestion, reaches it through the blood stream. The digestive enzymes produced in the pancreas are amylase, trypsin, and lipases. The amylase completes the break-down of carbohydrates, initiated by ptyalin in the mouth; the trypsin completes the digestion of proteins converting them into amino acids; and the lipases split the facts into their components, glycerol and fatty acids. Although the function of the pancreas is important, its digestive activities can, in an emergency, be carried on by the intestine—with slight loss of efficiency.

Early experiments indicated that alcohol increases the flow of pancreatic juice. However, some later studies by Brooks and Thomas (1953) demonstrated that "dilute alcohol has very little direct stimulating effect upon the volume or the enzymatic activity of the external secretion of the pancreas when instilled directly into the duodenum or given intravenously to dogs equipped with duodenal and gastric fistulas." These findings appear to indicate that wine or other alcoholic beverages stimulate the flow of hydrochloric acid directly, thus activating the pancreas secondarily. Dreiling and coworkers (1952) administered alcohol intravenously to human subjects without demonstrating any direct stimulation of the pancreas.

1812

Chalvon, G. ESSAI SUR LE VIN, CONSIDERE COMME CAUSE DE MALADIES, ET PRINCIPALEMENT COMME MOYEN THERAPEUTIQUE. *Paris: Thesis #143.*

An interesting essay recounting many attributes of wine but without supporting evidence. Among the answers to certain problems, the author offers quaint phantasies, such as: "Wine is the most natural beverage and the most salutary to man." In regard to the pancreas, he states: "Through sympathy, wine stimulates the liver and pancreas, augments their vital properties, develops and puts into action their functions." (pp. 10–11)

1903

Billings, John S. PHYSIOLOGICAL ASPECTS OF THE LIQUOR PROBLEM. *Boston and New York: Houghton, Mifflin and Company, 2 vols.*

"With wines, pancreatic digestion of proteids is more strikingly inhibited than by the stronger alcoholic liquors". . . Thus, a strongly acid wine, like a claret with only ten per cent of alcohol, has a far greater retarding action on pancreatic proteolysis than a sherry with twice that content of alcohol, but with less acidity." The author is in agreement with Sir William Roberts that, "When we consider how rapidly alcohol is absorbed from the stomach . . . we may consider that alcohol as used dietetically never interferes with tryptic digestion." (Volume I, p. 158)

1909

Pons, C., and Broeckaert SUR LA VALEUR ALIMENTAIRE DE L'ALCOOL. *Belgique Méd., 16:231–234.*

"Alcohol in small doses, as in wine, stimulates the pancreas to secrete its enzymes." (p. 231)

1910
McBride, C. A. THE MODERN TREATMENT OF ALCOHOLISM AND
NARCOTISM. *New York: Rebman Company.*

"If given in large quantities and concentrated, [alcohol]
diminishes the amount of gastric and pancreatic secretions; but
if given in small quantities and well diluted, it is said to increase the flow of secretions (Bernard and others). In large
quantities alcohol has a distinctly retarding effect on the activity of the salivary, gastric, and pancreatic ferments (W.
Hale White)." (p. 21)

1914
Babkin, B. P. DIE AÜSSERE SEKRETION DER VERDAUUNGSDRÜSEN.
Berlin: Julius Springer Verlag.

Referable to the pancreas, the author states: "Alcohol, introduced into the stomach, excites pancreatic secretion . . .
According to Gizelt, this stimulation does not occur if the
alcohol is introduced into the duodenum after the vagus nerve
has been cut." (pp. 283, 335)

1939
Mirsky, J. A., and N. Nelson INFLUENCE OF THE PANCREAS
AND THE LIVER ON THE OXIDATION OF ETHYL ALCOHOL. *Amer.*
J. Physiol., 127:308–314.

The rate of alcohol absorption into the blood in de-pancre-
atized dogs is observed and measured. It is suggested that insulin is not essential to the oxidation of alcohol and that when
a decrease in alcohol utilization does take place, after removal
of the pancreas, it is due to some factor other than the lack of
insulin *per se.*

1940
Beazell, J. M., and A. C. Ivy THE INFLUENCE OF ALCOHOL ON
THE DIGESTIVE TRACT. *Quart. J. Stud. Alc., 1:45–73.*

"Alcohol administered in moderate amounts and by any
route, . . . increases the secretion of pancreatic juice." (p. 69)

1944
Branch, A. PANCREATIC NECROSIS IN ETHYL ALCOHOL, METHYL
ALCOHOL AND ARSENIC POISONING. *Canad. Med. Ass. J., 51:*
428–430.

A discussion of the "most common poisons encountered in
human pathological states," namely, ethyl alcohol, methyl alcohol, and arsenic, and their effects on the pancreas. The

author states that these poisons "sometimes cause a very marked necrosis of the pancreas, a lesion which may cause death or at least may be a contributory cause . . . Whether the action is a direct one . . . is not certain." The discussion is based on personal observations made at autopsy.

1945

Weiner, H. A. ALCOHOL AND PANCREATIC NECROSIS. *J.A.M.A., 129:231.*

In view of the revival of interest in intravenous alcohol anesthesia, the author in a Letter to the Editor draws attention to the poorly understood and not widely known relationship between alcohol and pancreatic necrosis. Statistically, the relation is clear-cut, though unimpressive when compared to the total consumption of alcohol.

1952

Dreiling, D. A.; A. Richman, and N. F. Fradkin THE ROLE OF ALCOHOL IN THE ETIOLOGY OF PANCREATITIS: A STUDY OF THE EFFECT OF INTRAVENOUS ETHYL ALCOHOL ON THE EXTERNAL SECRETION OF THE PANCREAS. *Gastroenterology, 20:636–646.*

A report of a clinical study concerning the possible role of alcohol in the etiology of this disease. Twelve subjects were studied: 5 with and 7 without known disease of the pancreas. Secretin tests were carried out after a 12-hour fast; as a control, a 20-minute collection of duodenal secretion was obtained. Following the removal of the control material, a 5% solution of ethyl alcohol was administered intravenously to the point of drowsiness, sleepiness, giddiness and actual inebriation. From the results of this study, and keeping in mind other reports in the literature, the authors conclude that 1) the association of alcoholism and pancreatic disease is statistically significant; and 2) that intravenous administration of alcohol to the point of actual inebriation does not cause increased pancreatic secretion.

1953

Brooks, F. P., and J. E. Thomas THE EFFECT OF ALCOHOL ON CANINE EXTERNAL PANCREATIC SECRETION. *Gastroenterology, 23:36–39.*

A report of an experimental study in which the authors attempted to determine whether alcohol has a direct effect on pancreatic secretion or whether this could be due to gastric secretion secondarily stimulating the pancreas. Four dogs with duodenal and gastric fistulae were used; in one, subcutaneous transplant of the pancreas was carried out 9 months prior to the experiment. The solutions tested were: 10 cc. of 0.1% hydrochloric acid injected into the small intestine; 10 cc. of a 5% solution of 95% ethyl alcohol injected into the intestine; and a 5% solution of alcohol in physiologic saline. The results indicated "that the effects on the pancreas of drinking alcoholic beverages are not to be attributed to direct stimulation of pancreatic secretion by the alcohol . . . Insofar as stimulation of secretion is a factor in the harmful effects of alcohol on the pancreas it appears that the mechanism consists of primary stimulation of gastric acid secretion by alcohol and secondary stimulation of the pancreas by gastric juice as it enters the duodenum." (p. 38)

1957
Thompson, J. A.; J. R. Derrick, and J. M. Howard RELAPSING PANCREATITIS IN ALCOHOL AND NON-ALCOHOLIC PATIENTS. *Surgery, 42:841–845.*

1960
Walton, B.; H. Schapiro, and E. R. Woodward THE EFFECT OF ALCOHOL ON PANCREATIC SECRETION. *Surg. Forum, 11:365–367.*
Neither histamine nor alcohol, either orally or intravenously, stimulates pancreatic secretion if the stomach has first been removed. These findings suggest that the stimulation observed in the intact animal is caused by the flow of acid gastric juice into the duodenum with release of pancreatic secretion. The pancreatic juice obtained under these conditions resembles that produced by secretin.

1962
Walton, B. E.; H. Schapiro, and E. R. Woodward THE EFFECT OF ALCOHOL AND HISTAMINE ON PANCREATIC SECRETION. *Amer. Surg., 28:443–444.*
The augmentation of pancreatic secretion in dogs, observed in response to histamine and alcohol stimulation, is due to activation of the duodenal secretin mechanism rather than to any direct action on the pancreas.

1964
Sarles, H., and J. C. Sarles CHRONISCHE ALKOHOLISCHE PANKREATITIS. CHRONISCHE CALCIFIZIERENDE PANKREATITIS. *Verh. Deutsch. Ges. Inn. Med., 70:773–780.*

1965

Goodman, Louis S., and Alfred Gilman, editors THE PHARMA-
COLOGICAL BASIS OF THERAPEUTICS. *New York: The Macmillan
Company. Third edition.*

"Alcohol apparently has little deleterious effect on the intestinal or pancreatic functions. Digestion in the small bowel
is not likely to be impaired, perhaps because the alcohol reach-
ing the intestine is considerably diluted by gastric secretions
and mucus; and the secretion of pancreatic juice may actually
be stimulated by small doses of alcohol." (p. 146)

Goslin, J.; S. S. Hong; D. F. Magee, and T. T. White RELATION-
SHIP BETWEEN DIET, ETHYL ALCOHOL CONSUMPTION AND SOME
ACTIVITIES OF THE EXOCRINE PANCREAS IN RATS. *Arch. Int.
Pharmacodyn., 157:462–469.*

Rats given 15% alcohol to drink for six months, whether
fed ad libitum or iso-calorically with controls, were found to
have higher pancreatic protease and lipase than the water-
drinking controls. This was more obvious in those animals
receiving 18% protein than in those on the 6% protein diet,
In the ad libitum fed rats on the 6% and 18% protein diet,
alcohol increased liver fat above control levels, but less so in
the 18% than in the 6% protein group.

Ritter, U. ZUR ALKOHOLPANKREATITIS. *Deutsch. Med. Wschr.,
90:382–386.*

1966

Davis, A. E., and R. C. Pirola THE EFFECTS OF ETHYL ALCOHOL
ON PANCREATIC EXOCRINE FUNCTION. *Med. J. Aust., 2:757–760.*

Alcohol given intravenously to normal volunteers caused a
marked reduction in the volume of duodenal aspirate associated with normal or elevated concentrations of amylase and
bicarbonate. These effects were less pronounced when alcohol
was given intraduodenally. It was postulated that alcohol
causes pancreatic duct obstruction, and that this effect is related to the level of alcohol in the blood and not to the route
of administration.

Editorial ALCOHOL AND THE PANCREAS. *Lancet, 2:1353.*

Gamklou, R., and Y. Edlund ACUTE ALCOHOLIC PANCREATITIS
IN THE RAT. *Scand. J. Gastroent., 1:75–78.*

Pancreatic lesions were produced in rats by injection of dif-

ferent solutions into the pancreatic duct system. Bile containing about 1.5 mg. per cent alcohol caused more extensive
lesions (hemorrhagic necrosis) than normal bile. On the other
hand, 0.5 mg. per cent alcohol gave the same type of lesions
as did saline—interstitial edema only. Alcohol intake thus
appears to potentiate the injurious effect of bile on the pancreas. It was suggested that this might be an important factor
in the production of acute pancreatitis of alcoholism in man.

1967

**Maki, T.; G. Kakizaki; T. Sato; Y. Saito; T. Onuma, and N.
Noto** EXPERIMENTAL STUDY ON ALCOHOLIC PANCREATITIS. *To-
huku J. Exp. Med., 92:415–421.*

A limited experimental study on the rat fed 13% ethyl alcohol instead of water revealed significant elevations of serum
amylase, which was only partially rectified by a high-carbohy-
drate diet. Pancreatic edema was common, but fat necrosis,
ascites, or pancreatic necrosis was not observed at laparotomy.

Sarles, H., and C. Figarella ETUDE DE L'ACTION DE L'ETHANOL
ET DES GRAISSES ALIMENTAIRES SUR LE PANCREAS DU RAT. I.
VARIATIONS DES ENZYMES PANCREATIQUES (LIPASE, AMYLASE,
CHYMOTRYPSINOGENE, TRYPSINOGENE). *Path. Biol., 15:725–731.*

The authors have compared in Wistar rats the amylase, lipase, trypsinogen and chymotrypsinogen content of the pancreas in terms of protein and deoxyribonucleic acid in groups
of animals which were fed five different types of diet. At the
end of the 110-day experimental period the enzyme content
showed an increase proportional to weight increase, this difference being especially marked in the case of amylase and
less so in the case of the proteolytic enzymes. A diet moderately lacking in protein (7% casein) caused, in comparison
with the normal diet, a significant reduction in the amylase
content of the pancreatic gland. The reduction in lipase was
insignificant. There was no appreciable fall in the trypsinogen
and chymotrypsinogen content. With the 7% casein diet,
there was no difference in the enzyme concentration when the
fat intake was increased from 17% to 37% of refined arachis
oil. With a diet containing 7% casein, the inclusion of 20%
alcohol in the drinking water caused, irrespective of the fat
content, a significant decrease in the pancreatic concentration
of the four enzymes under study.

Davis, A. E. PANCREATIC FUNCTION IN ALCOHOLIC LIVER DIS-EASE. *Med. J. Aust., 1:508–509.*

The author emphasizes the high incidence of disturbances of pancreatic function in subjects suffering from alcoholic liver disease, especially cirrhosis of the liver.

1968

Burch, G. E., and A. Ansari CHRONIC ALCOHOLISM AND CARCI-NOMA OF THE PANCREAS. *Arch. Intern. Med., 122:273–275.*

The article discusses the relationship of chronic alcoholism and carcinoma of the pancreas, but not without prejudice. The data are scanty and the inferential conclusions transcend the evidence presented.

Chey, W. Y.; O. Kusakcioglu; V. Dinoso, and S. H. Lorber GASTRIC SECRETION IN PATIENTS WITH CHRONIC PANCREATITIS AND IN CHRONIC ALCOHOLICS. *Arch. Intern. Med., 122:399–403.*

The authors suggest that the frequent occurrence of hypo-secretion of acid or of frank achlorhydria in patients with chronic pancreatitis is related to the effect of the long-standing intake of excessive alcohol on the stomach.

Sardesai, V. M., and J. M. Orten EFFECT OF PROLONGED ALCO-HOL CONSUMPTION IN RATS ON PANCREATIC PROTEIN SYNTHESIS. *J. Nutr., 96:241–246.*

In a very well-designed experiment the authors demonstrate that there is a decrease in protein synthesis, including that of trypsin and ribonuclease, by the pancreas in animals fed an adequate diet and maintained on 20% ethanol as the sole drinking fluid. Control rats received the same diet with water ad libitum. Food intake determinations indicated that the effect on the pancreatic tissue was due to the ethanol *per se,* rather than any major alteration of caloric or protein intake.

Schapiro, H.; L. D. Wruble; J. W. Estes, and L. G. Britt PAN-CREATIC SECRETION STIMULATED BY THE ACTION OF ALCOHOL ON THE GASTRIC ANTRUM. *Amer. J. Dig. Dis., 13:536–539.*

A total of 17 experiments were carried out on 6 dogs. Perfusion of an antral pouch with ethanol increased the pancreatic volume and enzyme content after a 10–30 minute latent period. Gastric secretion also increased in each experiment, but after a 30–40 minute latent period.

1969

Med. World News DOES DRINKING PERIL LATE-STAGE FETUS? *Medical World News, December 26, 1969.*

At a symposium held at the Texas Research Institute of Mental Sciences, Doctors J. E. Idänpään-Heikkilä, W. M. McIsaac, B. T. Ho, and G. E. Fritchie revealed the persistence of high alcohol concentrations in various organs of the normal fetus, particularly in the pancreas, when beverage alcohol was ingested by the mother. Infusions of labelled ethanol into Rhesus monkeys demonstrated that during the early stages of the gestation, the ethanol in the process of metabolism was not heavily transferred to the fetus, but that in the later stages it was. The authors "guess" that the hypoglycemia of the newborn may be related to the accumulation of alcohol in the fetal pancreas due to the drinking of alcohol by the mother and by the inability of the fetus to metabolize the alcohol.

EFFECTS ON ABNORMAL FUNCTIONS

A review of clinical experiences with subjects suffering from pancreatitis reveals that the use of alcoholic beverages provokes distress, pain, and/or colic attributed to the stimulatory effect of alcohol on the secretions and cellular functions of the pancreas.

CONTRAINDICATIONS

The only major disease of the pancreas that is of significance at this point is pancreatitis. Since wine apparently stimulates the pancreas, even though indirectly, great caution must be used in permitting subjects of pancreatitis the use of wine. Where a pathologic condition exists, it is best that all beverage alcohol be prohibited. In general, then, wine is contraindicated in all diseases of the pancreas.

1946

Comfort, M. W.; E. E. Gambill, and A. H. Baggenstoss CHRONIC RELAPSING PANCREATITIS; A STUDY OF TWENTY-NINE CASES WITHOUT ASSOCIATED DISEASE OF BILIARY OR GASTROINTESTINAL TRACT. *Gastroenterology, 6:239–285; and 376–408*

An analysis of clinico-pathologic findings in a series of 29 patients with chronic relapsing pancreatitis without associated disease. The authors found that the onset of an acute attack was at times precipitated by "alcohol and dietary indiscretion," and that "in some instances a long history of alcoholism antedated the first acute seizure." They recommend that "since alcohol may be an aggravating factor in some cases, abstinence is advised." (p. 406)

7

An Epitome
of the Therapeutic Uses
# of Wine
in Disorders of the
Gastrointestinal System

In general, it may be said that small amounts of wine stimulate secretion of digestive juices while large, or excessive amounts, impede digestion by depressing secretion. One to three ounces of wine excites the appetite, two to four ounces stimulates salivary secretion. By this dual effect on appetite, as well as on secretion, wine stimulates the digestive function throughout.

In the stomach, wine promotes the flow of enzymes and hydrochloric acid—an effect said to be independent of the content of alcohol; while the tartrates, phosphates, and similar constituents act as buffers to perpetuate the flow of gastric juice over extended periods of time. The pancreas and certain other organs concerned with the production of digestive enzymes are stimulated secondarily.

Very small amounts of alcohol, per se, are known to stimulate intestinal peristalsis, perhaps due to the histamine-like action of the alcohol. A bactericidal effect, not due to alcohol, but to the content of colorless leucobase, has been reported. In recent years, an independent and broad bibliography on the antibiotic effects of the anthocyanins of wine has been published.

Wine facilitates the assimilation of nitrogenous substances, and stimulates deamination by the liver—sweet wines and dry white table wines being more active in this respect than red table wines.

In Latin countries, and especially in France, wine, often medicated, is used widely in the treatment of diseases of the digestive system, particularly anorexia, hypochlorhydria without gastritis, and hyposthenic dyspepsia. Minor hepatic insufficiency responds favorably to table wine, an observation rediscovered by modern clinicians. An important side effect of ingested white wine is the diuretic action on the kidneys in certain disorders of the urogenital system.

The anesthetic properties and the tannin content of wine make it a valuable adjunct in the treatment of colitis, spastic constipation, diarrhea and in certain infectious diseases of the gastrointestinal tract.

The nausea and vomiting of gastric irritation is alleviated by the use of effervescent wines or champagnes. This action is due to the anesthetic effect of carbon dioxide and the accelerated absorption of alcohol under these circumstances.

Moderately sweet wines are highly recommended because they are palatable stimulants of digestive function and offer analgetic effects as well as calories. The light aged red wines are beneficial, especially in convalscence and in geriatrics.

Some wines are best avoided—especially young or yeasty wines because they are fermentable, and highly alcoholized wines unless they are diluted, in which case they serve effectively when an increase in fluid intake is desirable.

Wine is contraindicated in any disease of the gastrointestinal tract characterized by hyperacidity, and when there are indications of potential hemorrhage, gastritis, pyloric stenosis, peptic ulcer, or cancer of the stomach. Because of its stimulating effect on the quantity and rate of flow of pancreatic secretion, wine is contraindicated in acute inflammatory disorders of the pancreas as well as in conditions associated with any dysfunction of the gallbladder and biliary tract.

For the guidance of clinicians who consider wine a desirable therapeutic agent, the following precepts are suggested:

1) Wine should be prohibited until a specific diagnosis is made and a logical therapeutic regimen can be instituted.

2) Wine, when indicated, should be prescribed in moderation for both its psychologic and physiologic effects.

3) Tonic wines should be taken on an empty stomach before the principle meals. Dietary alcoholic beverages and table wines are appropriately given with the dietetic prescription.

4) The dosage of wine should be gauged by the condition of the patient, the character of his illness, and the ultimate desired effect. From two to four ounces of wine—neat or diluted, according to indications—may be given with profit.

5) Wines should be discontinued upon the appearance of any symptoms of intolerance.

6) Because of the tranquilizing effect of table wines, they are helpful in keeping the obese patient on a restricted diet.

7) Alcoholic dietary beverages may react synergistically with tranquilizers, sedatives, narcotics and similar agents to reinforce the effects of these agents. When these agents are prescribed, dietary alcoholic beverages must be used with caution and control.

Index